## ADVANCE PRAISE

"In a world where intentionally safe spaces are often hard to find, Zabi [...]
a haven for letting out a deep breath and finally feeling truly seen. I [...]
gentle, practical yet nuanced, and so deeply validating. I am so touched by the thoughtfulness, fierceness, and tenderness that flow throughout this book, right alongside the incredible amount of research and practical tools available to the reader. This book reminds us that no matter who we are or what we've been through, healing is possible for all of us—and that there are so many accessible ways we can create a safer container for others who are on their own healing journey. *Trauma-Informed Yoga for Survivors of Sexual Assault* will be a profound and transformative offering for so many people."

—**Lisa Olivera**, therapist and author of *Already Enough*

"This book is wisdom gained from lived experience, rooted in fierce liberation politics, and compassionate to the core. Yamasaki illuminates countless assumptions made in the way that yoga is often taught—a methodology that pours further salt on the wounds that survivors come to heal. As a queer and trans survivor, this book is a balm; in anticipating my needs and experience, I can rest and feel whole. As a teacher, I have longed for this book for too long. Many trauma-informed yoga books do not attend to social injustice nor locate the author's positionality in systems of oppression. Yamasaki has all the references and relationships that I need as both a survivor and teacher doing work in social justice. Yamasaki offers up her own experience as a trauma worker and her intentional practices that allow that work to be sustainable while also illuminating how to adjust yoga practice to be specifically beneficial to survivors of sexual violence—and that same wisdom can be applied to so many of us directly impacted in various ways by the violence of this world."

—**Jacoby Ballard**, Yoga and Social Justice Teacher and Mentor

"This book means everything to me. And so does the author. As a woman of color I needed a voice I could finally identify with. Zabie Yamasaki is a true leader—transforming the culture of trauma recovery while transforming lives. 'Trauma-informed' is really *life*-informed. None of us leave here unscathed. We all carry pain onto our yoga mats, and with her guidance our mats can become safe havens for healing and transformation; Our yoga mats can be our way back home. We need this book. We need *her* book. Now more than ever."

—**Dr. Azita Nahai**, author of *Trauma to Dharma*

"Zabie Yamasaki has written a rare gift of a book that speaks to each reader with heartfelt compassion, profound mirroring, and unwavering respect. From the very first page we know we are in exceptionally capable hands, and provided with the safest, affirming, and embodied trauma-sensitive container in which to do deep healing work. She can guide the path because she lives it, and she is rooting for our aliveness with all her heart and brilliance. This book deserves to be in the canon of essential reading for survivors, providers, and practitioners of trauma sensitive yoga!"

—**Anjuli Sherin, LMFT**, author of *Joyous Resilience*

"*Trauma-Informed Yoga for Survivors of Sexual Assault: Practices for Healing and Teaching with Compassion* is a must for all yoga training required reading lists. Written with a depth of knowledge, care, and wisdom, this book bravely gives us access to healing tools and strategies to hold sacred space with awareness, responsibility, compassion, and understanding."

—**Tracee Stanley**, author of *Radiant Rest: Yoga Nidra for Deep Relaxation and Awakened Clarity* and *Empowered Life Self Inquiry Oracle*

"As a sexual trauma survivor, I found Zahabiyah Yamasaki's book *Trauma-Informed Yoga for Survivors of Sexual Assault: Practices for Healing and Teaching with Compassion* an incredible book that gives us the tools as yoga practitioners and teachers to foster self-acceptance and self-worth after sexual trauma through the yoga practice. This book helps us to serve our students in a thoughtful and embodied way. There are just so many ways we can apply yoga to our own healing and learning. Thank you for this incredible work which gives us so much insight into trauma-informed healing."

—**Dianne Bondy**, ERYT 500 at Dianne Bondy Yoga

"Zabie Yamasaki reminds us that trauma-informed practice is less about negotiating around the imprints of sexual trauma on our being, and rather, it is a centering of our humanity. For those who have survived the dehumanization of interpersonal violence, for those whose voices and bodies have been rendered invisible by individual and systemic forms of trauma—Yamasaki's invitation to recognize and honor our inherent wholeness is a counterbalance to pain that transcends language. In *Trauma-Informed Yoga for Survivors of Sexual Assault: Practices for Healing and Teaching with Compassion*, she offers the reader a pathway to reclaim their body through the holistic practice of yoga, allowing the site of profound violation to become a primary source of recovery."

—**Molly Boeder Harris**, Founder, The Breathe Network

"Zabie Yamasaki is finally taking the power of yoga and using it for good. This book is a missing link in the great reckoning that is happening within contemporary yoga and wellness spaces. We're finally addressing the needs of the most marginalized and those that have been abused. It is so refreshing to hear their stories and to consider how their concerns can be addressed so directly. I hope all yoga teachers read this book."

—**Jivana Heyman,** author of *Accessible Yoga* and *Yoga Revolution*

"This book is necessary reading for survivors and the people who tend to them. Zabie Yamasaki's offering is a healing salve to any of us who have experienced trauma, suffering, and hardship in our lives, which is to say: all of us. This book is medicine; it heals."

—**Dr. Allyson Pimentel**, Associate Director of Mindful USC and facilitator for UCLA Mindful Awareness Research Center and Insight LA

"In 2006, Tarana Burke started the #MeToo movement to support survivors of sexual violence, in particular black and brown girls, who suffer from sexual violence at three times the rate of white women and girls. In 2017 the #MeToo hashtag went viral when actress Alyssa Milano suggested in a Tweet that women who have been sexually harassed or assaulted respond by writing Me Too. Since then the #MeToo movement has expanded because sexual harassment and sexual assault impact people every day. The mission of the #MeToo movement is to connect survivors of sexual assault to the resources they need in order to heal. Now Zabie Yamasaki has provided a much-needed resource. Her book, *Trauma-Informed Yoga for Survivors of Sexual Assault: Practices for Healing and Teaching with Compassion*, offers a pathway toward healing the wounds of sexual abuse with trauma-informed yoga. An important read."

—**Gail Parker, Ph.D.**, CIAYT, psychologist, educator, and author of *Restorative Yoga for Ethnic and Race-Based Stress and Trauma* and *Transforming Ethnic and Race-Based Traumatic Stress With Yoga*

"*Trauma-Informed Yoga for Survivors of Sexual Assault* is a timely, powerful, and valuable resource for healing and empowerment. I can't recommend it more highly!"

—**Melanie Klein**, Empowerment Coach, Professor of Sociology and Gender/Women's Studies, cofounder of the Yoga & Body Image Coalition and coeditor of *Yoga & Body Image: 25 Personal Stories About Beauty, Bravery and Loving Your Body*

# trauma-informed yoga

## for survivors of sexual assault

✦

### Practices for Healing and Teaching With Compassion

# trauma-informed
# yoga

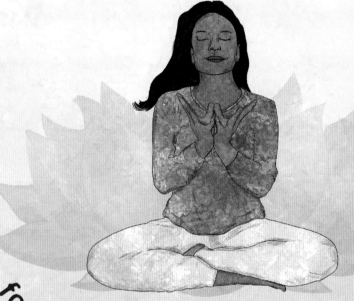

## for survivors of sexual assault

### Practices for Healing
### and Teaching With Compassion

**Zahabiyah Yamasaki, MEd, RYT**

Illustrations by Evelyn Rosario Andry
Foreword by David Treleaven
Foreword by Shena Young

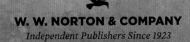

**W. W. NORTON & COMPANY**
*Independent Publishers Since 1923*

This book is a general information resource for current or prospective providers of and participants in trauma-informed yoga programs. It is not a substitute for medical or psychological diagnosis, treatment, or support for trauma survivors. If you are or may become a provider of trauma-informed yoga programs, please note that the programs, exercises, and guidelines in this book are intended to supplement, not substitute for, appropriate training, peer review, or clinical supervision. No technique or recommendation is guaranteed to be safe or effective in all circumstances. The author is not a lawyer and no suggestion in this book should be construed as legal advice. If you are or may become a participant in trauma-informed yoga classes, please consult your healthcare provider before starting any yoga program and please note that the instructions given for each yoga pose or exercise should be followed carefully, since even stretching can cause injuries if performed incorrectly. Any URLs displayed in this book link or refer to websites that existed as of press time. The publisher is not responsible for, and should not be deemed to endorse or recommend, any website other than its own or any content that it did not create. The author, also, is not responsible for any third-party material.

For information about permission to reproduce selections from this book, write to
Permissions, W. W. Norton & Company, Inc., 500 Fifth Avenue, New York, NY 10110

For information about special discounts for bulk purchases, please contact
W. W. Norton Special Sales at specialsales@wwnorton.com or 800-233-4830

Manufacturing by Versa Press
Book design by Molly Heron
Production manager: Katelyn MacKenzie

Library of Congress Cataloging-in-Publication Data

Names: Yamasaki, Zahabiyah A., author.
Title: Trauma-informed yoga for survivors of sexual assault : practices for
healing and teaching with compassion / Zahabiyah A. Yamasaki, M.Ed., RYT.
Description: First edition. | New York : W.W. Norton & Company, [2022] | "A
Norton professional book." | Includes bibliographical references.
Identifiers: LCCN 2021019765 | ISBN 9781324016137 (paperback) |
ISBN 9781324016144 (epub)
Subjects: LCSH: Rape trauma syndrome—Treatment. | Yoga—Therapeutic use. |
Mind and body therapies. | Psychic trauma—Alternative treatment.
Classification: LCC RC560.R36 Y36 2022 | DDC 616.85/210624—dc23
LC record available at https://lccn.loc.gov/2021019765
ISBN: 978-1-324-01613-7 (pbk.)

W. W. Norton & Company, Inc., 500 Fifth Avenue, New York, N.Y. 10110
www.wwnorton.com

W. W. Norton & Company Ltd., 15 Carlisle Street, London W1D 3BS

1  2  3  4  5  6  7  8  9  0

**TO MY HUSBAND, GARRETT, AND OUR SONS, GRAYSON AND HUDSON**

Thank you for loving me in my light and my dark, for being my greatest teachers, and for the gift of our collective resilience. I love you with all of my being.

**TO MY MOM, DAD, AND SISTER**

Thank you for your unconditional support and for reminding me that I am enough exactly as I am. Your love has carried me.

**TO MY INCREDIBLE FRIENDS, FAMILY, AND COMMUNITY OF SUPPORT**

There is not a day that passes that I take for granted how lucky I am to have your supportive presence in my life. Your inspiration has reminded me of all that is possible.

**TO EVERY SURVIVOR**

You are seen, you are valued, you are loved. You are worthy of your healing. You are worthy of your joy. Your story matters. You matter.

**ME, TOO.**

*Most of my life has been spent trying to shrink myself. Trying to become smaller. Quieter. Less sensitive. Less opinionated. Less needy. Less me. Because I didn't want to be a burden. I didn't want to be too much or push people away. I wanted people to like me. I wanted to be cared for and valued. I wanted to be wanted. So for years, I sacrificed myself for the sake of making other people happy. And for years, I suffered. But I'm tired of suffering, and I'm done shrinking. It's not my job to change who I am in order to become someone else's idea of a worthwhile human being. I am worthwhile. Not because other people think I am, but because I exist, and therefore I matter. My thoughts matter. My feelings matter. My voice matters. And with or without anyone's permission or approval, I will continue to be who I am and speak my truth. Even if it makes people angry. Even if it makes them uncomfortable. Even if they choose to leave. I refuse to shrink. I choose to take up space. I choose to honor my feelings. I choose to give myself permission to get my needs met. I choose to make self-care a priority. I choose me.*

> —DANIELL KOEPKE,
> ORIGINALLY PUBLISHED IN
> *DARING TO TAKE UP SPACE* (2020)

THIS BOOK IS FOR THOSE WHO HAVE KEPT THEIR STORIES RESIDING DEEPLY inside their bodies and for those who have shared. Those who might feel invalidated or marginalized. Those who are unable to share due to reasons of safety or fears of not being believed. Those who feel the power of their bravery and courage building, and those who need reminders of their light. Those who need to see and feel their identities and experiences affirmed and reflected. I will continue to fight for you and do my part to recognize and validate the scope of healing from sexual violence and the spectrum of emotions we carry far beyond the initial trauma(s). You are worthy of support that is tailored to your unique and nuanced needs, and you are a part of a community of resilience that is keeping you held and lifted at all times. You are not alone.

# Contents

# A Note Amid the Pandemic

I share the words that follow in this book as a gift from my heart, from my experience and journey as a survivor, and as a resource for healing and doing healing work with integrity, compassion, and nuance. This book was birthed amid the pandemics of COVID-19 and racial injustice. And I hope it serves as a reminder that you are never alone in your experience. That there is a community that is surrounding you and keeping you lifted in even the most isolating of times. Remember that your light shines even in the dark.

I never imagined the grave and heartbreaking conditions that would surround the world as I wrote this book. There were so many days that I felt helpless and wanted to hibernate, yet I also found profound and pivotal moments where I was feeling so much that I needed to move it from my body to pen and paper. I could feel the shifts and the lightness. Those moments sustained me and gave me an outlet to process and cope with big feelings.

I think this book was meant to take shape within a messy and nonlinear timeline because in many ways it mirrors the healing process and it unearthed resilience in ways I hadn't yet had a language for. And as my dear friend and author Dr. Azita Nahai says, "Let's face it, if we were signing up for easy, we wouldn't be here—humaning our way through this life—constantly braving our way through the new, the unfamiliar, and the uncertain" (@azitanahai, Instagram, April 27, 2020).

This book is a combination of personal narrative, survivor truths, supportive guide for those passionate about trauma-informed yoga, fierce yet tender lens of advocacy, and soft place to land for survivors. I always say that **showing up is the hardest part**. So I invite you to take a moment to send yourself compassion for everything it took to get to this very moment. Honor your capacity. Honor your beautiful existence. Honor your strength. We are learning every day that we can do hard things. And your body and your survival strategies should not be shamed for the ways they have protected you. For the hyperarousal moments that kept you safe. And for the constant cues for rest that it inevitably sends.

I hope this book can be a healing balm, a place of refuge and retreat, and a container for all you may be holding. Thank you for trusting and traveling this journey with me. It is an honor to have you hold this book in your hands and your hearts.

# Foreword

This book has the power to change lives. It offers a road map for trauma-informed yoga at a time when we desperately need it, and it's written by someone who embodies the principles she teaches. I know this from experience.

I met Zabie Yamasaki when she hosted me in her role as program director of Trauma-Informed Programs at UCLA. I'd published a book on trauma-sensitive mindfulness a year earlier and she'd invited me to address her community. I arrived a bit early and watched Zabie and her team register people as they began to trickle in.

I was amazed by what I witnessed. Zabie greeted everyone by name, asking personal questions about their family and specific questions about their work. Her introduction later that morning wove personal stories with contemporary research, holding the audience rapt. I quickly realized that Zabie wasn't just a trauma-informed yoga teacher. She was a visionary leader in her community who genuinely cared for those she led.

Like many, I've been imploring Zabie to write this book for years. In her eyes, trauma-informed approaches are an essential part of yoga and meditation. They are not just a specialized niche. Zabie is passionate about helping trauma survivors practice yoga, and empowers teachers to do just that.

Yoga is something of a double-edged sword when it comes to trauma. While many trauma survivors will benefit from yoga, the intense focus on sensations can also be dysregulating. Intrusive thoughts, memories, and painful sensations can intrude into consciousness at any time, leaving those struggling with trauma susceptible to dysregulation, dissociation, and retraumatization in practice.

Zabie reminds us this isn't something to fear but to be prepared for. Yoga practice often won't cause trauma, but it can reveal it. As yoga teachers and practitioners, we can be ready to respond skillfully when trauma arises. We can incorporate Zabie's teachings into our toolkit and be more confident in our approach.

Inside of this, working with survivors of sexual assault requires sensitivity and skill. To understand sexual assault is to understand the social dimensions of trauma—the collective denial that survivors can encounter, for example, or the shame that often accompanies traumatic wounds. Like all trauma, sexual assault does not occur in a vacuum. It's connected to the world around us. And Zabie continually turns us towards this fact to empower our teaching.

Ultimately, this book is about empowerment. Each chapter is born out of Zabie's experiences of what works (and what doesn't) in trauma-informed yoga for survivors of sexual assault. You're about to learn powerful tools that you can adopt right away in your teaching and practice. There's a refreshing practicality with Zabie's writing, and innovative teachings born out of trial and error.

I'm thrilled you've found this book. It couldn't have come at a better time, nor from a more powerful teacher and human. May it bring healing and transformation to us all.

DAVID TRELEAVEN
AUTHOR OF *TRAUMA-SENSITIVE MINDFULNESS:*
*PRACTICES FOR SAFE AND TRANSFORMATIVE HEALING*

MAY 2021
SAN FRANCISCO, CALIFORNIA

# Foreword

I have a good friend named Shy, one of my favorite people on the planet. The first time I said "I love you" we were parting ways after having some sweet quality time and in preparation for our week. In the overwhelm, she managed to utter "Thank you" and scurried to the nearest exit. Some days passed and we found ourselves revisiting the moment. I learned about her relationship with love and discovered that "I love you" was foreign and also "too common" to capture what lived between us. Instead she offered, "I am happy you exist." This happened some years ago, long before I met Zabie. I've since adopted this sacred acknowledgment and embrace as an expression, a love story, and in this moment, a rare offering. To my beloved friend, teacher, colleague, and sister-healer—Zabie, I am happy you exist.

It is an honor to stand in this opening and new beginning, in healing, for so many that will be touched by this book. My name is Dr. Shena Young. I am a licensed body-inclusive psychologist, trauma-informed educator/yoga teacher, reiki master, healer, & survivor of many things. I own a private practice, Embodied Truth Healing & Psychological Services, an intimate and intentional space for seeking truth and healing, mind, body, heart, and spirit. My work centers the lived experiences of my beloved Black, Indigenous, & People of Color (POC) communities, the stories that are captive in their bodies, and the traumas wedged between generations.

I've lost the memory of how Zabie and I met some years ago, but our first interaction was a long phone call and we were smitten with what we discovered. It seems we had been living in our respective corners of the world, birthing kindred visions, and were divinely guided into concentric overlap. To discover another woman of color doing *this* work felt like a nostalgia you hope will linger.

What a magical moment to be here, basking in the lingering. This book is at once a memoir, an invitation, and an opportunity . . . in healing. Zabie truly poured herself into these pages, undeniably guided by her resilient ancestors and spirit guides, and the wise healer inside that has journeyed survivorship. This is what happens when a being knows why they came into this world—they journey, they bring medicine, they imprint, and they leave the world better than they found it, in the way only they can.

It is a consecrated crossroads that many survivors stumble upon, where their pain and purpose meet one another. May this book meet you at the intersections of holding yourself and the survivors you love and care for. Zabie has written a comprehensive guide that facilitates deeper understanding of the relationship between sexual trauma and the body. She beautifully ambassadors the imminent movement toward trauma-informed care as the standard we are all so deserving of. In these pages, we learn to listen to the voice of the body, to appoint it as the elder healer, to remember what it knows, and to entrust our healing to the ageless wisdom of yoga. In these pages, we learn to relinquish control of other people's narratives, to cue remembrance of choice, to affirm generously; we return to the breath, and we invite reclamation of home in the body. These are the healing reparations my beloved communities of color are worthy of, for embodiment to be encouraged and fortified, boundaries respected, and nervous systems to be restored to calm.

As you journey forward in healing and in these pages, may the words of my sweet and gentle friend Zabie be close by. "I invite you to turn the volume of your heart all the way up and the volume of your thoughts all the way down." May anyone who reads these pages be compelled to heal, to expand, and to transcend.

DR. SHENA YOUNG (SHE/HER/HERS)
LICENSED BODY INCLUSIVE PSYCHOLOGIST
TRAUMA INFORMED EDUCATOR/YOGA TEACHER
EMBODIED TRUTH HEALING & PSYCHOLOGICAL SERVICES
@EMBODIEDTRUTHHEALING

JANUARY 2021
LOS ANGELES, CALIFORNIA

# Introduction: Transcending Sexual Trauma through Yoga

*"Never have I felt so safe without having to speak a single word about my assault."* I'll never forget the day when a survivor shared these words with me after participating in an 8-week trauma-informed yoga series for sexual assault survivors. Every part of her was beaming. I think that is the power of survivors gathering in circles to share community, connect in their truth and the power of their stories, move and breathe at their own pace, and celebrate the choices they have with their own bodies. As she accessed safety in the space, her capacity for connection also increased. It was a defining moment for me in the scope of my work. And a powerful reminder of the need for this body-based modality to be accessible to all survivors and integral to the services that are offered to survivors at universities, trauma agencies, rape crisis centers, and clinical settings across the country.

I have witnessed something so moving by offering this practice from a trauma-informed lens: Survivors—of all gender identities, racial and ethnic backgrounds, sexual orientations, and abilities—can finally feel and believe with every part of their bodies that their trauma does not define them. The practice is a reminder of their innate capacity to heal and that they are never alone in their experience. I still remember the very first trauma-informed yoga series that I taught, nearly 10 years ago. I remember the butterflies. I remember the passion. I remember the pathways for healing that suddenly became possible. I began teaching trauma-informed yoga classes in the community for many reasons. To support survivors in what is oftentimes a lifelong process of healing. To create spaces in which to love ourselves throughout the journey and be reminded that our pain is not invisible. To affirm that we are not broken and that we can return to our bodies on our own terms. To support empowerment and empathy and space in which to be seen. To foster compassion when we tap into the deep knowing that there may be no sense of finality to this thing called healing. To hold on fiercely to our worthiness amid the many storms we will navigate in this life. To let ourselves be present with moments of relief and of joy. To consciously practice self-love with the many paradoxes of healing and hurt, courage and fear, grief and joy. To know that there are many entry points to healing.

Yoga can be a pathway for the integration of mind, body, and spirit amid all of the disintegration that trauma causes. This notion alone has been a guide and anchor for me in my own healing and as I pursued my passion for creating affirmative and inclusive healing spaces. My work has been an intersection of my worlds as a survivor, a woman of color, and a trauma-informed educator and yoga instructor. Because of the impact that trauma has on the body's physiology, I feel that we do a huge disservice to survivors by leaving the body out of treatment. I've learned this firsthand doing direct work with survivors and having the honor to witness their courage and resilience and hear their stories.

Yoga is an ancient practice that began in India and seeks to help people transcend suffering. As Susanna Barkataki, shares, "Yoga has always had a perspective of seeking to heal trauma and alleviate inner and outer anguish" (@susannabarkataki, Instagram, September 9, 2020). In Sanskrit, the term *Ahimsa* (which is one of the five yamas of the eight-limbed path of yoga) means "nonviolence." And as an emotional practice, this has anchored me deeply in the scope of my work with survivors. I knew that I wanted to build a program that spoke to the language of the body and honored the roots of the practice. A program that was soulful, intersectional, accessible, and culturally affirming at its core. I believe that in the context of our various professional roles we have an obligation to be mindful of the way that trauma manifests for our students. For yoga teachers this would mean offering the same care and attention to experiences of trauma that we do to physical injuries. We have a powerful opportunity to support survivors in their recovery, offer them restorative tools to manage their stress response, help them gently unpack trauma imprints and support the flow of energy throughout their nervous system, and most importantly: **help them access safety in their own bodies**. I believe that one day every trauma agency, university, hospital, recovery center, rape crisis center, and domestic-violence shelter will offer trauma-informed yoga as an integral part of treatment and services for survivors. I also think it is critical that we normalize trauma-informed frameworks being integral to yoga teacher trainings.

Trauma-informed yoga is an empowering yoga practice that prioritizes the lived experience and healing of each and every student. Safety, trust, choice, and control are some of the core components of the practice. The frameworks of trauma-informed yoga that will be explored in this book include empowerment-based language, supportive presence and the embodied practice of holding space, self- and community care for the teacher, consent-positive assists, safety of the physical space, trauma-sensitive breath work, sensitivity to triggers, and cultural considerations and accessibility. Trauma-informed yoga is a unique and effective way to help survivors heal. The practice can help survivors safely reconnect to their bodies, allowing them to access resources when they are ready. Through our research at the University of California, survivors shared that the practice decreased their symptoms of PTSD, anxiety, and depression; helped them develop positive coping strategies; empowered them to seek out additional support resources to prioritize their mental health; and helped them practice self-compassion, among many other benefits.

All of my professional roles have entailed facilitating presentations on trauma. And after every presentation I have facilitated, a number of survivor disclosures have followed. In my numerous conversations with survivors over the years, I have noticed some consistent themes. One has been a need to feel something tangible. So many survivors have shared that they continue to live with and navigate the debilitating trauma symptoms that permeated their lived experience, long after the incident(s) occurred. They voiced so openly and vulnerably about wanting to manage the somatic symptoms and triggers that were arising in their bodies every single day. Another theme that has frequently arisen is that many survivors are not quite ready to process their experiences through talk therapy. They have shared that it did not feel like an accessible option for them. According to Forge and the Transgender Sexual Violence Project (2015)

> . . . few victims received professional emotional support soon after they were assaulted. Only 14% got help within the first week, with another 19% getting help within the first 6 months, and an additional 10% getting help before the first year was up. However, 57% did not receive their first professional emotional help until more than a year after the assault(s), with 28% not receiving help until ten or more years after they were assaulted.

Additionally, navigating life in the aftermath of sexual assault can already feel like a largely invisible experience, which can lead to further isolation. This demonstrates the critical need to broaden the scope and spectrum of healing to be intentional and nuanced far beyond the initial experience(s) of trauma. In one campus implementation of the trauma-informed yoga program, 40 survivors submitted interest forms to participate. Of those 40, only 10 were currently connected to the counseling center or survivor advocate. The other 30 survivors indicated that the yoga program was their first entry point in receiving any type of help or support related to their trauma(s).

We are at a defining moment in our world, where survivors are boldly speaking their truth as a result of Tarana Burke's inspiring movement, #MeToo. She founded the movement in 1997 to center the sexual assault experiences of Black and Brown girls, whose stories have been historically and heartbreakingly silenced and minimized. The #MeToo movement has paralleled the trauma-informed yoga movement for some time now, and now more than ever there is a powerful convergence of the two. Stories live inside the bodies of survivors, many of whom are not able to vocalize their experiences for a multitude of reasons, such as for their own safety or because they hold marginalized identities. Additionally, if there is one thing that the year 2020 revealed and woke the world up to, it is the staggering and devastating racial disparities that have permeated every aspect of our society. Not only has COVID-19 disproportionately impacted communities of color, but the unfathomable violence against Black bodies is something we cannot turn away from. Black lives have always mattered.

Trauma-informed care, which will be further explored in Chapter 1, has always been rooted in anti-oppression and antiracism frameworks. The practice is incomplete without acknowledging the intersections of survivor identities, racial injustice, and the cultural trauma that is far too prevalent in our world. The antiracism movement and the sexual violence movement have never been separate. There is no checklist. And trauma work was never meant to be rushed or unpacked quickly. This work will entail a life-long commitment to making systemic policy change, doing inner work, pursuing growth, being intentional and thoughtful as service providers, centering the identities of survivors who are most vulnerable, affirming that we cannot do anti-sexual violence work in isolation, acknowledging when we do not know the answers, sitting with discomfort, and listening and learning. Our nervous systems are a profound guide in leading us toward a more just world. And most importantly, survivors of color deserve a deep space for belonging, and healing modalities that acknowledge and affirm their beautiful existence.

Sexual violence impacts all aspects of human functioning: the physical, mental, behavioral, social, and spiritual. And for years the anti-sexual violence movement has been limited in resources and scope of practice, offering a narrow range of services for survivors to access support in the healing process. Molly Boeder Harris shares:

> After the advocacy in the Emergency Room, when the community support group stops meeting or for those who never had the opportunity or the safety to say the words "I was raped" aloud, where do survivors turn next as they navigate this (sometimes) lifelong journey of healing? (Boeder Harris, 2013)

The spectrum of what healing looks like is so vast. While each survivor's healing process is unique—due to factors such as cultural barriers, access to health insurance, financial accessibility, and stigma around seeking mental health services (to name just a few)—it is essential that service providers and support agencies for those who have experienced sexual violence offer multiple pathways for survivors to heal (and are provided with the resources needed to make their work sustainable). Something that must always guide our work: **Not every survivor will heal in the same way; they are all worthy of a menu of options that put them at the center of their own experience.**

This book aims to provide a foundation for how to offer yoga to survivors of sexual assault in a safe, effective, evidence-based, and healing way. Drawing upon the framework of trauma-informed care and trauma-informed yoga program development and curricula, while weaving in my own personal narrative and inspiring survivor stories, this book explores practical considerations for yoga teachers, mental health professionals, educators, activists, healing professionals, and survivors who are interested in integrating trauma-informed yoga into the scope of their work and/or healing. The guidance in this book aims to fill a gap in service delivery for survivors by providing trauma-informed education at its intersection with yoga. In the pages that follow you will find a comprehensive and supportive guide to healing as well as to working mindfully and compassionately with the sensitive, nuanced, and intentional needs of survivors of sexual assault.

## From My Heart to Yours

*Stress and trauma can disconnect you from yourself. It's beautiful to see you making your way back home.*
—DR. THEMA BRYANT-DAVIS

There are so many days I reflect on the journey that my organization Transcending Sexual Trauma Through Yoga has taken me on. The years of healing. Of work. Of unpacking messages that didn't belong to me.

Of refusing to believe those who tried to diminish my voice. Of relentless tears. I remember the moments they have led me to. The power of being grounded in my inherent worth as a survivor. The softness that self-compassion brings when imposter syndrome makes me want to shrink. The joy that comes with fiercely believing in my dreams and watching them unfold. The palpable feeling of bravely taking up space despite all the ways trauma makes it easy to feel small. I remember that not one part of this journey has been easy. But finding purpose amid the pain has fulfilled me in ways I could never have imagined. It is amazing what can happen when we give ourselves permission to fully step into our own truth, worth, power, belonging, and joy.

I frequently return to the stacked journals on my bookshelf that are filled with my preparations and writings for trauma-informed yoga classes over the past decade. I get emotional seeing the handwritten notes I made to myself, the folded page corners, the quotes and passages that resonated with me, the faded covers holding wisdom and reminders, the ebbs and flows of grief, and the reminders in healing. They have the ability to take me right back to where I was during that particular chapter of my journey. They reveal so much of what my heart was holding.

Each day this beautiful community reminds me of the power of showing up, even on my hardest days. Because more than anything, the survivors I've been honored to meet on this journey have been my greatest source of strength. Thanks to all who believed in this little dream. Your support has held my heart through some of the hardest moments of my life. And I'll never forget it. We don't just need community; our entire physiology depends on it to thrive. We were never meant to do this alone.

I have had the greatest honor of being witness to the most remarkable experiences of resilience in my career. Working with survivors of sexual assault has been one of the greatest gifts of my life. Being witness to the human experience and our capacity to move through, despite the unimaginable, is a strength that exists all on its own. Survivors embody the intersection of soft and fierce. And when survivors build programs for survivors, I believe that some of the most powerful work and healing unfold. Because these programs are built from the markers of lived experience and create an unspoken bond that is grounded in the meaning of "survivor-centered."

My sincere hope is that this book is a reminder to you that your dreams and your healing are absolutely possible. Never let anyone tell you that you are not capable of doing anything you have ever envisioned for yourself in this life. You are worthy of it all and your voice is so needed. Because if there is one thing the world could benefit more from—it is an abundance of healing.

## Disclaimers

*Caring for myself is not self-indulgence. It is self-preservation, and that is an act of political warfare.*
—AUDRE LORDE

*Anyone who is interested in making change in the world also needs to learn how to take care of herself, himself, theirselves.*
—ANGELA DAVIS

Perhaps you picked up this book because you are a yoga instructor who wants to gain tools for creating a safe and comfortable environment for your students. You might be aware of the high percentage of trauma survivors who are taking your classes every single day. Maybe you are a therapist who wants to incorporate trauma-informed yoga into your clinical practice. You may be a survivor who is looking for healing, support, affirmation, and connection. Whatever the reason that brought you to the moment of holding this book, my heart is just so grateful you are here. As you move through these pages, I hope that it feels like a soft and supportive place to land. I hope that you read words and participate in practices that speak to the wisdom of your body and soothe your heart. There are a few things I would like to share to support you in working toward an embodied sense of safety as you engage with the material in this book.

At the level of our psychobiology, our nervous system is constantly communicating to us about our needs. And trauma has a tendency to challenge both our internal and our external sense of safety in the world. I want to support you in creating a strong container as you start to process and integrate the material you learn as a survivor, for your clients, for your students, and/or for those you hold space for. I am acutely aware that many of us come to this work with our own experiences of trauma. This requires us to be extra gentle with ourselves. It is a constant reminder that we don't have to have it all figured out. That we cannot intellectualize our way out of the healing process. That we can take all the time we need. That our own healing can coexist with the healing of those we serve. That our resilience, the language of our nervous system, and our messy pathway to post-traumatic growth can be our greatest gift in holding space for others. This is your permission to be compassionate with yourself when reading material that may be activating or triggering. You are invited to take pauses. To go slow. To listen to your body. To skip to some of the trauma-informed practices that are offered in Chapter 6. There is absolutely no rush.

On a daily basis we are constantly consuming information that leads to balance or imbalance in our lives. This could be through the media and news we consume, our stressors, racial trauma, triggers we are processing, the relationships and environments that surround us, family dynamics, internal and external pressures we may be experiencing, our places of work, our circumstances, the identities we hold, or many other challenges that impact our lives in ongoing ways. This may also be compounded with our own lived experience of navigating life after trauma. So much of moving through this material will be about honoring your story, your needs, your feelings, your care, and your unique healing journey. It might also mean allowing yourself to feel moments of relief, joy, and peace and to remind yourself that **you are so deserving**.

I would like to shift the paradigm of me in the role of teacher and you in the role of student. As Nikki Myers, founder of Yoga of 12-Step Recovery, says, "there is no hierarchy in healing" (personal communication, June 8, 2013). This is a concept that has always anchored me in trauma-informed work. There is no one-size-fits-all approach when it comes to trauma healing. And we are certainly not having uniform experiences.

We are unique and powerful beings, holding our own stories inside our bodies, and traveling the journey of our intersecting identities of race, ethnicity, class, gender identity, orientation, ability, mental health, age, language, and religion, among many others. Your story and your experience are valid. And if we were together for an in-person trauma-informed yoga training, I would likely be drawing a box on a large sheet of paper. I want to invite you to not get too stuck in the learning box. In many instances, folks come to my trainings wanting a template and checklist for how to be more trauma informed and/or wanting a specific set of asanas for healing trauma. And while I will certainly share some broad considerations around trauma-informed care at its intersection with yoga, there is no checklist, shortcut, or yoga posture that could ever capture the complexity, nuance, and sensitivity of this work. Instead we do our very best to provide survivors with a menu of supportive options that honor the roots of the practice, empower them to decide what feels best for their healing process, support them in celebrating the beautiful choices they have with their own bodies, practice humility in moments when we may cause harm, and hold ourselves accountable toward repair.

Being trauma informed is a philosophy and a systemic framework of the way we truly see people and honor their humanity. It is a lifelong commitment to leaning in and doing the work of being an ally, educating ourselves, being aware of our biases, and engaging in culturally affirming practices. It is committing to and engaging in our work that at all costs avoids retraumatization. It helps us to compassionately and empathetically hold a safe container. And it allows every interaction to be a powerful reminder: **Survivors are the experts of their own experience**.

Finally, I hope that the tools in this book allow you to approach your healing and your work with survivors in renewed ways. I hope you begin to see that your own self-care and your own mental health are integral to doing this work from a safe, embodied, and nurturing lens. Burnout has never been a badge of honor and we were never meant to do trauma work in unresourced ways. In leading a centering practice, Prentis Hemphill said, "We can ground but it doesn't mean we do not act. We are not looking for a practice that is going to take us out of engagement with the world . . . but rather to be with what is" (@prentishemphill, Instagram, June 17, 2020). I hope that the tools inspire your activism, revolutionize your work and your healing, and remind you that rest is a radical practice.

> **Rest is deeply personal and looks different for each of us. Below are some supportive invitations to explore:**
> - Postponing or cancelling something on your calendar when you are having a hard week.
> - Delegating. It is okay to not be the one taking the lead all the time.
> - Taking a mental health day.
> - Asking for a phone call vs. another video call or keeping your zoom camera off.
> - Unapologetically saying "I don't have capacity."
> - Unfollowing social media accounts that trigger you.
> - Taking a full lunch break not in front of a screen.
> - Honoring your cues of exhaustion. Knowing when it is time to turn down the chatter of the outside world and the urgency of others and return to yourself.
> - Reminding yourself often that you may not get to everything on your list and that is okay.
> - Leaving the dishes in the sink, the laundry in the basket, the toys on the floor...
> - Releasing the pressure to respond to everyone else's sense of urgency (e-mails, texts, social media). Honoring the urgency for rest.
> - Setting limits on how often you engage with trauma related material.
> - Choosing a restorative yoga class over a more active one.
> - Exploring not checking your phone upon waking and letting the outside world impact your mood before you even wake up.
>
> *(list continued on next page)*

*(list continued from previous page)*

- Sitting down in nature, resting your gaze, and listening to the sound of your own breath.
- Being discerning with what you say yes to.
- Assessing your bandwidth and capacity at the beginning of your week and being selective with scheduling and intentional with restorative time.
- Taking a midday nap.
- Being okay with saying "I rested" when someone asks you what you did.
- Showing up authentically.
- Honoring your value and your boundaries.
- Protecting your energy, time, and space.
- Not over-explaining yourself.

## RESOURCING TOOLS

I spend a lot of time thinking about the ways in which we take in trauma-related material (news, media, trainings, books). It may feel helpful to have a self-care plan in place as you engage with material that might be triggering to you. If it feels supportive, you might want to have some resourcing materials around you or ideas for increasing your comfort as you move through the book. These might include:

- A blank journal for processing your own feelings and emotions as well as space in which to integrate your learning
- A resourcing corner in your home (comfy blanket, lavender, candle, etc.)

*(list continued on next page)*

*(list continued from previous page)*

- A yoga bolster, pillow, blanket, or any additional props to increase your comfort and safety and/or to use in the sample practices. You are invited to flip to the trauma-informed practices shared in Chapter 6 to pause, move, and rest.
- Essential oils
- Fidget toys
- Affirmation cards
- Pipe cleaners
- Coloring pages, colored pencils, or other art supplies
- Calming music
- A trauma-informed meditation or guided visualization that feels safe
- Grounding exercises
- Breaks for fresh air
- Nourishing snacks and hydration
- An emotional-safety ritual
- Connecting with a therapist or support system
- Or anything else that would support you when engaging with trauma-related material. Remind yourself that you don't have to take in all the material in one sitting. Give yourself time and grace.

## Guidance for Interacting With This Book

As you can see, this book is intended for multiple audiences, including survivors, yoga instructors, mental health and other healing professionals, and staff at universities and trauma agencies who would like to integrate this modality into their scope of services. Throughout the book I have clarified the focus of the material, so please feel free to skip around to the sections that feel most relevant to you and your needs at any given time.

**Part One of this book focuses on understanding the trauma-informed lens and is broken down into four chapters:**

CHAPTER 1: **The Neurobiology of Sexual Assault and Trauma**

This chapter provides an accessible and survivor-centered lens of the neurobiology of sexual trauma and why integrating the body is a critical component of trauma healing. Specific references highlight the "window of tolerance" (Siegel, 1999), the nervous system, the somatic impact of trauma on the body, and the healing elements of the vagus nerve (Porges, 2017). The chapter also covers common symptoms that survivors of sexual assault may experience in the aftermath of trauma, and discusses the nuance of embodied inequality and race-based trauma, the physiological imprints of trauma, trauma triggers, the impact of trauma on the brain, dissociation, and the somatic experience of PTSD.

CHAPTER 2: **How Trauma-Informed Yoga Supports Healing**

This chapter highlights personal survivor narratives as well as data on the impact of the 8-week trauma-informed yoga program. This chapter also defines the elements of trauma-informed care (safety, trust, choice, collaboration, empowerment, and cultural competence [National Sexual Violence Resource Center 2017]) and "the four Rs" (Realizes, Recognizes, Responds, and Resists retraumatization [Substance Abuse and Mental Health Services Administration, 2014]). Specific references are made to the grassroots history of trauma-informed care and the work of Black and Brown feminists who were on the front lines putting survivors at the center of their own experience. Additionally, a foundation will be provided for trauma-informed care as a philosophy and way of being in the world, as opposed to a checklist.

CHAPTER 3: **Teaching Trauma-Informed Yoga**

This chapter covers the following frameworks for teaching from a trauma-informed lens: (1) empowerment-based language, (2) supportive presence and the embodied practice of holding space, (3) self- and community care for the teacher, (4) consent and physical assists in yoga spaces, (5) creating safety in the physical yoga space, (6) a trauma-sensitive approach to breath work and mindfulness (7) supporting students who are triggered, and (8) cultural considerations and accessibility. The frameworks are taught from a broad perspective to be applicable to multiple professionals who would like to implement elements of this modality into the scope of their work.

CHAPTER 4: **Dear Survivors, Your Body Remembers. Be Gentle With You.**

This is a special chapter dedicated to the resilience of sexual assault survivors and is a tribute to their lived experiences. It is an affirmation of survivors' stories, a reminder of the wisdom they hold in their bodies and of their innate capacity to heal. It serves as a dedication to all those who are holding their experiences with constriction and looking for more ease, space, and safety within.

**Part Two of this book includes two chapters that focus on implementing trauma-informed work as a professional and also provides a tool kit of practices and affirmations for healing:**

CHAPTER 5: **Comprehensive Guidance on How to Create a Yoga Program for Survivors**

This chapter covers the following core frameworks for yoga teachers, clinicians, educators, and other healing professionals who are interested in building a curriculum and starting a trauma-informed yoga program for survivors of sexual assault: (1)

creating buy-in from a university/trauma agency, (2) presenting powerful visuals and communicating your message, (3) utilizing the power of collaborations, (4) working with mental health professionals, (5) identifying your audience and building an intake process, (6) building a curriculum, (7) marketing and outreach, (8) understanding assessment and liability, and (9) honoring your voice. I have successfully implemented the trauma-informed yoga curriculum at roughly 30 large institutions and trauma agencies (e.g., Yale, Stanford, Johns Hopkins, UCLA, and USC, to name a few). This chapter will serve as a powerful "how-to" implementation guide for readers and a resource for those looking to take theory to practice.

CHAPTER 6: **Trauma-Informed Yoga Tool Kit and Affirmations**

This chapter serves as a supportive place for survivors to learn affirmations that are coupled with trauma-informed yoga practices for integration into the healing process. This chapter is also an informative reference point for yoga instructors, mental health professionals, educators, and other healing professionals who are looking for guidance on practices and tangible tools to share with survivors in classes, workshops, or clinical practice.

# trauma-informed yoga

## for survivors of sexual assault

✦

Practices for Healing and Teaching
With Compassion

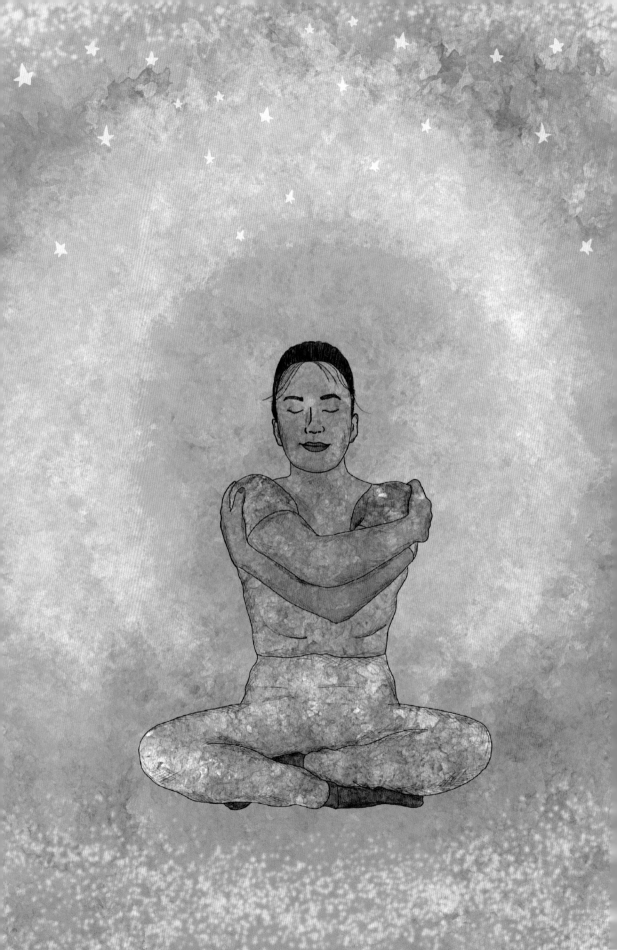

PART ONE

# Understanding the Trauma-Informed Lens

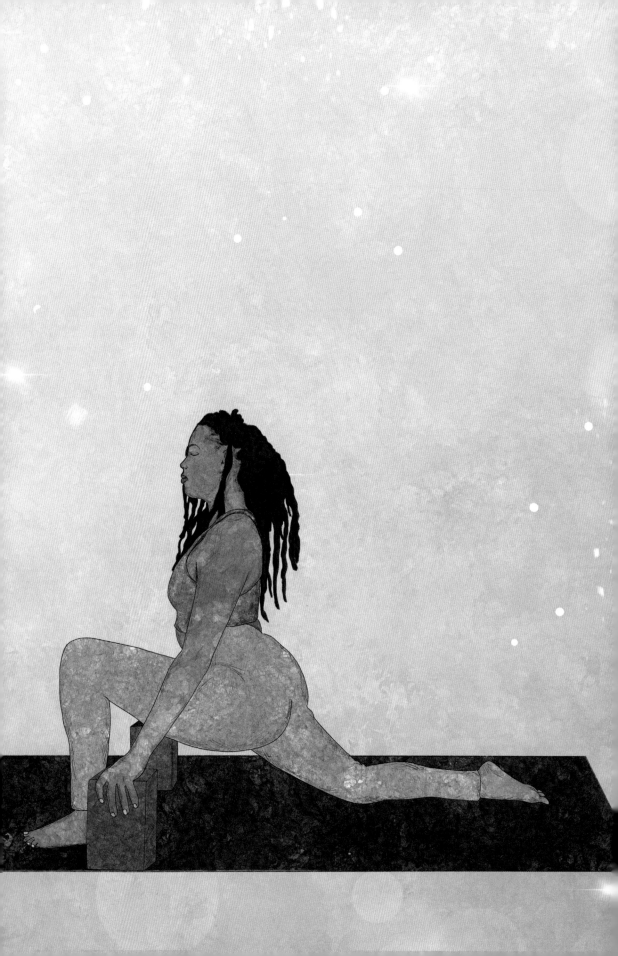

# ✦ 1 ✦

# The Neurobiology of Sexual Assault and Trauma

*Trauma has roots not just in the mind, but also in the body. Pain can be trapped in the body in a way that the mind can't easily reach, let alone discharge.*
—BO FORBES, *YOGA FOR EMOTIONAL BALANCE*

A trauma is an event that is monumental in its impact on the body. It is an event, series of events, circumstances, or accumulation of experiences that are life-threatening, cause extreme fear and distress, and can impact one's physical, emotional, mental, social, and spiritual sense of safety in the world. These experiences can overwhelm our capacity for coping. Trauma is also subjective and based on the lived experience of each and every individual. What is traumatic to you is traumatic to you. Your story is important. Your feelings are valid.

## What Does "Trauma-Informed" Mean?

*In a victim-centered approach, the victim's wishes, safety, and well-being take priority. Victim-centered feminism would bring to bear specialized services, resources, cultural*

*competence, and ideally trauma-informed perspectives*
*toward caring for the needs of those who go through the*
*trauma of testifying or pressing charges or filing lawsuits.*
*We would provide a conduit to the professionals best*
*able to assess survivor needs, and we'd provide critical*
*support to survivors in the aftermath even if they were not*
*eligible for traditional victim-support services that may*
*exist in their area. These skills are imperative to building*
*rapport and trust with survivors, meeting their needs, and*
*assisting them in creating a sense of safety and security in*
*their lives. . . . We need to understand that sometimes the*
*fiercest warriors need care and kindness.*
—MIKKI KENDALL, *HOOD FEMINISM*

The term "trauma-informed" often gets thrown around as a buzz-word. It's important to me to share what the term means, where it comes from, and how it can be applied to multiple settings within the scope of our work and healing. Experiences of "trauma influence how survivors approach and respond to services, which is why it is critical for service providers who are working with sexual assault survivors to recognize the various expressions of trauma and acknowledge and affirm the role that it plays in their lives" (NSVRC, 2017). Trauma-informed care also means honoring all of a survivor's various intersecting identities, including age, gender identity, socioeconomic status, ethnicity, nationality, sexual orientation, immigration status, employment, body size, physical and mental illness, and disability, to name a few. This impacts how they move through the world, who they feel safe with, who they trust, the identities that are most salient for them, and who can effectively hold space for them.

Trauma-informed care originates from the constructs of trauma theory which state that traumatic memories can be stored as physiological reactions to stimuli that recall the traumatic experience if the memories are not processed (Reeves, 2015). Trauma-informed care can be considered a framework for understanding survivors of trauma (But-ler et al., 2011). Primarily, "to be trauma-informed is to understand the involvement and impact of violence and victimization" and to not com-mit further harm (Butler et al., 2011, p. 177). Additionally, researchers state that creating trustworthiness, promoting empowerment (Butler et al., 2011), inspiring hope (Cleary & Hungerford, 2015), emphasizing strengths, and engaging in cultural competence (Elliott et al., 2005) are additional elements of trauma-informed care. The National Sexual Vio-lence Resource Center (2017) presents the following core frameworks of trauma-informed care:

- *Safety*
- *Trust*
- *Choice*
- *Collaboration*
- *Empowerment*
- *Cultural Competence*

The ultimate goal of trauma-informed care is to support the healing and growth of survivors and, at all costs, to avoid retraumatization. Its underlying philosophy is actually grounded in grassroots and survivor-centered models that stem from early rape-crisis-center and domestic-violence movements. The framework was built from the powerful work of Black and Brown feminists who were on the ground doing direct work with survivors of violence, addressing their nuanced and culturally spe-cific needs, and putting them at the center of their own experience. The Substance Abuse and Mental Health Services Administration (SAMHSA, 2014) shares, "It has become evident that addressing trauma requires a multi-pronged, multi-agency public health approach inclusive of public education and awareness, prevention and early identification, and effec-tive trauma-specific assessment and treatment." SAMHSA has provided a helpful framework of approaching trauma-informed care through the four R's:

REALIZES: the widespread impact of trauma and understands potential paths for recovery

RECOGNIZES: the signs and symptoms of trauma in clients, families, staff, and others involved in the system

RESPONDS: by fully integrating knowledge about trauma into policies, procedures, and practices

RESISTS: retraumatization (SAMHSA, 2014)

What makes the framework so powerful is that it understands the impact of trauma not only on survivors but also on communities and on those that hold space for survivors. As a result it works to build healthy and resilient organizations that contribute to collective and community care. There is a quote by Rebecca Remen (1996) that always lands on my mind, body, and soul every time I read it: *The expectation that we can be immersed in suffering and loss daily and not be touched by it is as unrealistic as expecting to walk through water without getting wet.* This is a gentle reminder to all those who work in social-justice and trauma fields: **Your mental health matters. You matter.** The systems in which we work are only *truly* trauma informed if they intentionally and compassionately support a holistic culture of care.

We need administrators and leaders to prioritize the mental health, resilience, well-being, and workload of educators, therapists, yoga instructors, advocates, and others who work in a variety of helping professions (especially since a large number of those professionals are survivors themselves). What frequently ends up happening is a parallel process in which the harm we are trying to prevent and heal plays out systemically in our work environments and creates its own cycle of violence. I will share more about this concept in Chapter 3, but for now I just want to share that creating compassionate environments and policies for service providers is integral to trauma-informed care.

According to Rebecca Macy and colleagues (2018), a number of service providers who work with individuals who have experienced trauma (e.g., abuse and assault, human trafficking, military combat, natural disasters, and terrorism) "have expressed growing interest in the potential benefits of yoga to help their clients and patients cope with the effects of trauma, including trauma-related mental illnesses such as anxiety, depression, and posttraumatic stress disorder (PTSD)." This has been evident through the growing interest of clinicians seeking continuing educational opportunities related to trauma-informed yoga. What has also been so meaningful about this growing movement and interest is the support and holistic care it provides to service providers and the ways it reenergizes and reengages them in their work.

Finally, and most importantly, we must consistently examine the systems of oppression that make it challenging for survivors and service providers to thrive. Trauma Aware Care shares, "If we focus solely on nervous system regulation and self-healing, but don't acknowledge and work to change systemic oppression, we are missing a fundamental piece of the puzzle" (@traumaawarecare, Instagram, January 8, 2021). This is integral to our lifelong journey as trauma-informed practitioners in truly serving all survivors, honoring and affirming their intersecting identities, and acknowledging and fighting against the systems that create barriers to access care.

## PREVALENCE OF SEXUAL ASSAULT

Trigger/Content Warning: I want to invite you to opt out of this section if reading about a high incidence of sexual violence might be triggering to you. Please know you are not alone in your experience. If you choose to continue, please take your time and go slow. All of your feelings are welcome here.

Sexual assault is one of the most psychologically damaging crimes that a person can experience. And the numbers speak volumes. Seventy percent of adults in the United States have experienced some type of traumatic event in their lives; that's 223.4 million people (The National Council for Behavioral Health, 2013). As reflected on the RAINN website (rainn.org), every 73 seconds, an American is sexually assaulted (Department of Justice, 2019). The National Intimate Partner and Sexual Violence Survey (Black et al., 2011) estimates that approximately 53.2 million women and 25.1 million men in the United States have experienced some form of sexual violence over the course of their lifetime. That's 78.3 million women and men in the United States alone. Transgender and nonbinary individuals experience sexual violence at even higher rates. According to the 2015 U.S. Transgender Survey (James et al., 2015), almost half (47 percent) of transgender individuals have been sexually assaulted at some point in their lifetime. The numbers are even higher for communities of color, as according to the U.S Transgender Survey Report on the Experiences of Black Respondents, 53 percent of Black respondents have been sexually assaulted in their lifetime and 13 percent were sexually assaulted in the past year (James, et al., 2017). According to the statistics on the RAINN website, Native Americans experience the greatest risk of sexual assault, as American Indians "ages 12 and older experience 5,900 sexual assaults per year." Incidents of sexual violence in the military are staggering and often go unreported, yet the DoD estimates that 20,500 service members experienced sexual assault in 2018 (rainn.org). According to a meta-analysis of 80 other studies conducted by Walker and colleagues in 2019, almost half (47.9%) of survivors of child sexual abuse were revictimized later in life. It is estimated that "80,600 inmates each year experience sexual violence while in prison or jail" (RAINN.org).

Many survivors who navigate their lives in the aftermath of trauma may live in constant fear of revictimization. In this time of #MeToo, even more survivors are feeling empowered to share their stories and are looking for support as they navigate the triggers that may be lingering in their bodies long after the assault(s) occurred. I want to invite you to take an inhale in at your pace, and exhale out in your way. Start to take note of how this information lands for you in your body. You may be noticing strong internal sensations or overwhelm. It is okay to take a break. Take all the time you need and return to the material whenever you feel ready.

There has been increased scrutiny specifically on college campuses since the release of the Dear Colleague letter in 2011 that came from the Obama administration (U.S. Department of Education, 2011). This was a revolutionary initiative that led to the White House Task Force to Protect Students from Sexual Assault. The task force announced a series of actions to help combat the problem of sexual violence on college campuses, including getting clarity around its prevalence and scope, comprehensive prevention efforts, guidance on responding effectively and supportively to survivors, and more transparency around the federal government's efforts to enforce policies (White House Task Force to Protect Students From Sexual Assault, 2017). As a result, institutions across the nation have been consistently forming task forces and coalitions and taking a serious look at their current sexual assault policies, protocols, and services to reevaluate and refocus their efforts to support survivors and ensure campus safety. But we will always need more than a task force to create systemic change and profoundly shift the culture that perpetuates sexual violence.

We have seen a resurgence in this movement over the past several years due to Chanel Miller (2019) courageously sharing her story of surviving the assault of Brock Turner; the moving and powerful testimony of Christine Blasey Ford; the Harvey Weinstein trial and his being sentenced to 23 years in prison; the advocacy and attention around the national epidemic of backlogged and untested rape kits; revised guidelines on Title IX recommendations from the Trump administration and his appointees (though unfortunately these were not trauma informed and they reversed a lot of protections for survivors); and the groundbreaking work of California's first surgeon general, Dr. Nadine Burke Harris, to screen every student for childhood trauma before entering school. Finally, we will never forget the courageous story of Oluwatoyin "Toyin" Salau, an inspiring 19-year-old activist who fought for justice for all Black lives and centered queer and trans Black lives in her activism. She was a survivor who also lost her life. She will be remembered for her brave heart and compassion. We will continue to fight for her.

Sonya Renee Taylor shared these powerful words, which have been etched in my mind as we think about the various systems of oppression that pervade all levels of our society:

We are not being asked to reckon with **one** system. We are being asked to reckon with every single system of oppression that seeks to disconnect us from our own humanity. Seeks to disconnect us from the humanity of others. Seeks to oppress and power over. Seeks to find itself through the degradation and violence of other bodies. Every entity, every structure, every system that defines itself in that way is being asked to fall. (Sonya Renee Taylor, @sonyareneetaylor, Instagram live, June 16, 2020)

Sexual assault is a public health crisis. It impacts all of us. And it requires communities, policymakers, government officials, educators at all levels, survivors, healers, mental health professionals, and social-justice and survivor advocates, among many others, to work collaboratively and through a trauma-informed and healing-centered lens, for change to permeate all levels and for survivors to be granted the dignity; support; and holistic, inclusive, and lifelong care they deserve.

## The Physiological Impact of Trauma

*When we begin to understand that much of what we think of as "symptoms" are actually survival strategies, we make space for compassion and healing.*
—DR. JENN HARDY, @DRJENNHARDY, INSTAGRAM, JULY 6, 2020

*The body says what words cannot.*
—MARTHA GRAHAM

We cannot compartmentalize the way that humans experience trauma. Trauma impacts all aspects of our being. The experience of sexual violence often elicits feelings of intense fear and powerlessness, and can flood and overwhelm a survivor's nervous system and internal capacities. Many survivors report feeling a loss of power and control as a result of the violence they have experienced. When seeking support through the trauma-informed yoga program, survivors have shared with me so much of what they are holding, including feelings of disconnection, dissociation, and isolation; experiences of self-blame; lack of trust; and overwhelming minimization of their feelings and experiences, to name a few. They have shared their struggles related to accessing resources that help them address the impact of trauma on their bodies, complicated family dynamics, challenges around articulating or sharing their story, lack of safety, barriers to seeking support such as holding marginalized identities or faith-based concerns, and their deepest hope for healing and community that they carry in their hearts.

According to a study by Reeves (2015), somatization of trauma occurs when traumatic memories are tied to physical sensations in the body. Additionally, experiences of trauma can result in post-traumatic stress disorder (PTSD), depression, hyperarousal, conditioned fear responses to trauma-related stimuli, loss of trust and hope, and social avoidance (Macy et al., 2018; Telles, 2012). Rebecca Campbell's research confirms that rape survivors can experience physical health distress, and the somatic imprints of sexual trauma can significantly disrupt their nervous system (Campbell et al., 2003). This can manifest as hyperarousal, including anxiety, fear, intrusive memories, hypervigilance; and hypoarousal, which includes emotional numbing, social avoidance, fatigue, low energy, and dissociation (Emerson & Hopper, 2011). Trauma is often a somatic reaction. Survivors sometimes register their trauma not as stories but as felt physical sensations in their bodies. Many survivors experience a range of physical symptoms in the aftermath of trauma, including:

- chronic pain
- dysregulated breathing
- throat constriction
- rigid body posture
- lack of presence
- nervousness
- gastrointestinal symptoms

*(list continued on next page)*

*(list continued from previous page)*

- overworking
- sweaty palms
- heart palpitations
- flashbacks
- anxiety
- insomnia
- heightened sensations
- clenched muscles (neck, shoulders, jaw)
- sunken chest, heavy heart
- aches and pains (headaches, backaches)
- migraines
- numbness
- self-harm
- eating disorders
- shortness of breath
- dissociation
- gynecological issues
- muscle tension

These visceral experiences in the body are often a result of the vagus nerve disengaging. The vagus nerve plays an instrumental role in the expression of emotions in our body. The vagus nerve is our 10th cranial nerve, and when we feel safe, the ventral branch of the vagus nerve supports our ability to feel and access rest and calm. It supports survivors in understanding their inner landscape, especially the interconnection between their gut and their emotional state. Pat Ogden refers to the visceral sense as enteroception, which "tells us about the movements occurring within our internal organs, such as racing of the heart, butterflies in the stomach, nausea, hunger or that 'gut feeling'" (Ogden et al., 2006). All of these symptoms should also be held through a culturally affirming lens, as a survivor's various intersecting identities can impact their lens, their lived experience of trauma, and their access to safety and resources in the world.

Dr. Shena Young specializes in the impact of trauma on the chakras and she shares how the chakras are "energy stations that hold genetically coded memories that are both psychological and physiological in nature" (Young, 2020). The "*chakras* contain bundles of nerves and major organs as well as our psychological, emotional, and spiritual states of being" (Shah, 2020). There are seven chakras: Root Chakra (Muladhara), Sacral Chakra (Swadhisthana), Solar Plexus Chakra (Manipura), Heart Chakra (Anahata), Throat Chakra (Vishuddha), Third-Eye Chakra (Ajna), and Crown Chakra (Sahasrara) (Miller, 2004). When we experience imbalances in these energy channels, it can lead to physical symptoms, chronic pain, and other types of illness. The body remembers and our stories are visceral. The practice of trauma-informed yoga has inspired so many possibilities within the realm of healing and mental health. It is an evidence-based mind-body modality that supports survivors in managing a variety of psychosomatic symptoms, strengthening their enteroceptive capacity, building neuroplasticity and vagal tone, and enhancing their overall health, well-being, and resilience. Trauma-informed yoga often helps survivors build incremental shifts over time to widen their window of tolerance, strengthen their coping skills, and, most importantly, feel empowered in their choices and grounded in their worth.

We must also consider the complexity of trauma, in that it encompasses not just experiences of sexual trauma (or other types of trauma) but also the added layer of trauma due to systemic racism. We cannot address sexual violence without also having intentional and nuanced conversations that address how various forms of oppression contribute to sexual violence and who is at risk. This requires us to be very thoughtful about the intersection of racism, discrimination, bias, and prejudice. I remember attending a bystander intervention training in which the facilitators were discussing specific ways to intervene in situations where violence might occur. What felt particularly distressing to me was that there was no mention of looking through the lens of race. With her voice shaking, one participant asked them about the biases that people hold when thinking about whether or not they believe someone is worthy of intervening for (with reference to the lived experiences of people of color). Sadly, they looked at her with blank stares.

When someone is being oppressed, this can manifest in the body as a trigger or as physical sensations, similar to PTSD. This is known as embodied-inequality or race-based trauma (Carter, 2015). Dr. Gail Parker discusses how yoga is a practice that helps people of color to experience safety in their vulnerability. This is often a new experience for folks who have a daily accumulation of racial stress. She shares in such moving ways that people of color need the therapeutic experience of resting safely. They need a pathway to understanding what the "absence of stress" feels like in their bodies (Parker, 2019). This is why it is critical to be continually rooted in anti-oppression frameworks, ancestral wisdom, and Indigenous healing practices when teaching trauma-informed yoga. We must hold intentional spaces for experiences of racial trauma and the ongoing impacts this has on the nervous systems of people of color.

Trauma, at a very primal level, can make rest an incredibly challenging concept for survivors. When we teach trauma-informed yoga, integrate this modality into the scope of our work, or have the opportunity to practice it, we give survivors a space where they can begin to gently unpack what rest means for them. The hope is that rest can ultimately feel restorative and safe, instead of taking the form of numbing, dissociating, avoiding, or suppressing. These are all common symptoms of trauma, and for many of us, they are survival strategies. I do want to share that the protective nature of hyperarousal (something one of my mentors Molly Boeder Harris writes beautifully about) can be a profoundly healing concept to reflect upon and integrate, as it is never my intention to create shame around the survival strategies that have kept us safe. Jessica Maguire says, "A healthy nervous system is not always calm. It's flexible and resilient" (Jessica Maguire, @repairing_the_nervous_system, Instagram, May 12, 2020). This entire journey of unpacking the ways we have survived and continue to survive requires extra gentleness and care.

Healing from sexual assault can be a lifelong and nonlinear journey. The residue of the trauma can stay with us and linger in the body long after an assault occurs and can manifest as a trigger. A trigger is a

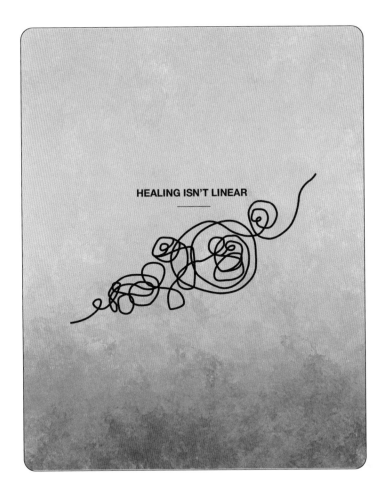

HEALING ISN'T LINEAR

physiological response outside of a survivor's control that reminds them of a past experience of trauma. If a survivor is undergoing extreme stress, if they have a flashback or a nightmare, if they run into their perpetrator, if they smell a certain perfume or cologne, if a yoga teacher places hands on them without their permission, they can suddenly be placed right back in that experience of trauma as if it were happening in that moment. Andrea Papin writes, "Anything that reminds us of a previous danger can activate our physiology" (personal communication, June 2019). These words are simple, yet profoundly describe what happens when a trigger takes place.

When I am triggered, it typically takes the form of a flashing hot feeling in my belly that moves its way up to my face and ultimately signals to my body to shut down or freeze. My body is communicating to me that my current environment or circumstance is not safe. When a survivor experiences a trigger, they may be responding to the present moment as if it were the past. Their body may be misreading the cues of what is happening in their current environment, and the threat feels very real. These moments deserve so much compassion, as they can bring us right back to the visceral memory of the trauma. Even if the rational brain is communicating, "I am safe," the emotional lower brain does not believe it is safe.

Jenn Wooten shares this:

> In the wild, when an animal is threatened and it cannot fight the threat, it freezes and becomes immobile. This response is governed by the dorsal vagal complex of the parasympathetic nervous system. In a freeze response, the nervous system largely shuts down all unnecessary functions. Breathing becomes shallow. The life force wanes. Pain and all other sensation becomes numb. Or the opposite, pain and inflammation heightens as our bodies respond to the surging levels of cortisol. (Jenn Wooten, @wakingyoga, Instagram, September 16, 2020)

Many of us continue to push through and function through these states. The year of 2020 was one of the most visible examples of this, yet many survivors have been functioning in this way for a lifetime, given the ongoing impact of trauma on their lives. Emily and Amelia Nagoski, authors of *Burnout*, discuss the concept of "completing the stress cycle," which refers to working through the accumulation of stress in the body and the various ways this manifests physiologically. They share, "Most of us are walking around with decades of incomplete stress response cycles . . . just waiting for a chance to complete" (Nagoski & Nagoski, 2019).

As shared previously, during trauma, the nervous system can become incredibly activated when we experience a trigger or have a recollection of a trauma memory. Even if the threat is not real, it can *feel* very real. It can send our bodies into states of hyperarousal where we may experience increased sensations, anxious thoughts, feelings of threat or fear, flooded emotional reactivity, hypervigilance, and panic. Sigh. Living in constant states of hyperarousal is so incredibly exhausting and can lead to adrenal fatigue. Our adrenals regulate the levels of cortisol in our bodies and adrenal fatigue can occur when our system is working in excess. This can ultimately lead to chronic fatigue, which in the context of trauma can make even seemingly small tasks feel incredibly overwhelming and fatigue inducing. If this is a feeling that is familiar for you, please know that you are not alone. You deserve to rest. Our bodies are not designed to be in constant states of hyperarousal. The way this can manifest in the body is by sending us into states of hypoarousal (depression, lethargy, isolation, dissociation, and numbing). Adrenal fatigue occurs when our system is working in overdrive and our "surge capacity" is depleted. Dr. Ann Masten defines surge capacity as a "collection of adaptive systems—mental and physical—that humans draw on for short-term survival in acutely stressful situations" (Haelle, 2020). What many survivors navigate is chronic and impacts every aspect of their lives. When you feel tired, it can mean so many different things. **Tenderness, compassion, community, intentionality, and rest are all integral components of trauma healing.**

## THE EMOTIONAL IMPRINTS OF SEXUAL ASSAULT IN THE BODY

It is critical for service providers and those holding space for survivors to recognize the various expressions of trauma and the ongoing impact that trauma can have on a survivor's life. This impacts who they feel safe with, who they trust, and the nuance involved in the holistic services needed throughout the trajectory of their healing. In her article "Releasing the Tangles of Trauma Through Body-Energy Healing," Jen Altman (2007) shares that "losing touch with our bodies also affects the way we view the world and our ability to respond to future challenges: we may become anxious, hypervigilant, withdrawn and isolated, less confident, less trusting, and more fearful." Trauma-informed yoga can support survivors with addressing a range of these symptoms at their pace and in their own unique and tailored way.

In yogic philosophy, trauma causes something called vasanas. Vasanas (also known as residual feelings) are essentially emotional imprints that live in the body in the aftermath of trauma. They often get deep rooted, hardwired, or lodged in various areas of the body, depending on the nature of what someone has experienced (Criswell et al., 2014). This can impact our nervous system, endocrine system, and physiology and can lead to physical symptoms and illness. These symptoms are often somatic reenactments of the various traumatic experiences that survivors have gone through and the coping skills they have had to rely on to access safety.

Trauma-informed yoga can help survivors gently tend to embodied trauma imprints and bring them to the surface. And with greater awareness, time, and patience, survivors often feel empowered with new tools to name and address their symptoms and survival responses and identify ways to work through them. This can ultimately lead to a space where survivors can expand their capacity for neuroplasticity and take powerful steps toward post-traumatic growth. The term "post-traumatic growth," first coined by Calhoun and Tedeschi in 1999, refers to our capacity to heal and includes "relating to others with greater compassion; finding new possibilities, personal strength, spiritual change, and a deeper appreciation of life" (Rozentsvit, 2016).

Dr. Azita Nahai, author of *Trauma to Dharma*, says (2018), "When we spend all our time looking outside ourselves for answers, we move farther and farther away from where they already reside—inside." So as you continue on this journey, remember the profound wisdom your body holds. I think some of the greatest gifts we can offer one another are reminders of our innate capacity to heal and of the fact that we are not defined by our trauma(s). We will continue with this topic in Chapter 2.

## A Closer Look at the Impact of Trauma

*I don't know of one thing I don't fear. I fear getting out of bed in the morning. I fear walking out of my house. I have great fears of death . . . not that I will die someday, but that I am going to die within the next few minutes. I fear anger . . . my own and everyone else's, even when anger is not even present. I fear rejection and/or abandonment. I*

*fear success and failure. I get pain in my chest, and tingling and numbness in my arms and legs every day. I almost daily experience cramps ranging from menstrual type cramps to intense pain. I just really hurt most of the time. I have shortness of breath, racing heart, disorientation, and panic. I'm always cold, and I have dry mouth. I have trouble swallowing. I have no energy or motivation, and when I do accomplish something, I feel no sense of satisfaction. I feel overwhelmed, confused, lost, helpless, and hopeless daily. I have uncontrollable outbursts of rage and depression.*
—PETER LEVINE, *WAKING THE TIGER*

What do you notice within your own body when you read these words? Many survivors share with me how compromised their sense of safety becomes when trying to distinguish safety from danger or intuition from trauma. That sense of hypervigilance that may accompany the way we move through the world in the aftermath of unfathomable violence to the body. I will never forget when I had the great honor of hearing Tarana Burke speak about the journey that led her to "Me too." She talked about how surviving sexual violence can oftentimes feel like a very invisible pain and experience as others cannot see the broken pieces that survivors may carry internally (personal communication, April 22, 2019). This offers important insight into the lived experience of a trauma survivor and what they might be holding on any particular day. This also gives us a sense of the type of physical or emotional energy they may be carrying with them to their yoga mat and the ongoing experiences that may impact their sense of safety and trust.

Survivors of sexual assault often share that they feel victimized not only by the assault but then again by the system. They are frequently asked to recount and share concrete details of their story to multiple people (law enforcement, service providers, campus officials, friends and family, medical professionals, and others). And they often report that they do not feel believed. Survivors may experience a range of victim-blaming statements, which can have a detrimental impact on their inner states, leading to an accumulation of trauma residue. In many cases this internalization of traumatic experiences, feelings, and emotions can elicit trauma symptoms (the vasanas that we discussed earlier). This adds to the layers of emotional trauma they may already be experiencing, including self-blame, lack of trust, lack of control, fear, minimization of experiences, isolation, and what I think can be the most damaging, which is this notion that it is not okay to feel the way they feel.

Two common victim-blaming questions that survivors often hear are "Why didn't you run away?" and "Why didn't you fight back harder?" You may frequently hear the concept of the fight-or-flight response; only recently have we heard more about the concept of "freeze." Freezing happens in nearly 50 percent of rape cases; in the context of sexual assault, it is referred to as tonic immobility or rape-induced paralysis (Heidt et al., 2005). This is when during an assault a survivor becomes physically frozen and unable to move. This may occur because of debilitating fear that they may be further harmed. When survivors hear the questions mentioned above, it completely minimizes their experience and makes them feel that they could have done more to prevent the assault from happening to them—leading to further minimization of their overall experience.

I invite you to take a moment and rest a palm over your heart and over your belly if that feels comfortable for you. Perhaps explore taking an inhale in and an exhale out. Explore your breath at your pace. If it feels available, you could explore neck rolls, extending your arms up to the sky, or bringing your palms to the back of your shoulders for a self-massage. If the tears come, let them come. Take a moment to pause and continue reading when you feel ready. There is no rush to your healing and your learning. **You are believed. You are supported. You deserve to take all the time you need. Healing is not linear.**

## THE PHYSIOLOGICAL IMPACT OF PTSD

PTSD may take the shape of arousal, numbing, avoidance, and vigilance. And in many ways, dissociation is the essence of trauma. It is characterized as a strategy to leave the body because oftentimes trauma has overwhelmed a survivor's nervous system and it is too painful to be present with those sensations. The experience is overwhelming in that thoughts, physical sensations, sounds, images, emotions, and sensory information all related to the trauma trigger start to take a course of their own. For people who have PTSD, a flashback can occur at any time, whether they are awake or asleep. The experience is unpredictable and terrifying. PTSD is the body's way of communicating that we have undigested sensory residue that wants to be processed. According to the Sidran Institute, 1 in 13 people in the United States will develop PTSD during their lifetime.

If you are a yoga instructor or a mental health professional integrating this modality into your work: Being predictable in your presence, sequences, and practices is so important when working with survivors

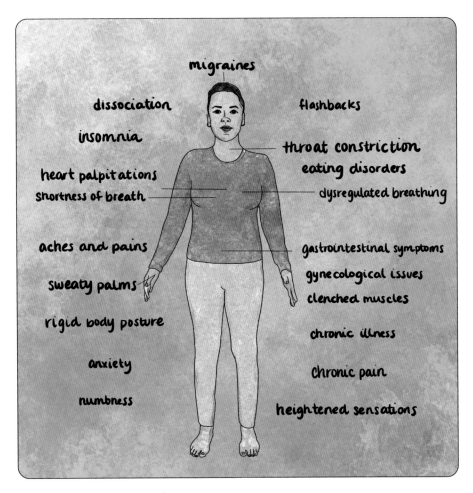

The Somatic Impact of PTSD

who have PTSD. When teaching trauma-informed yoga, consistency and repetition may help support and stabilize a survivor who is struggling with a dysregulated nervous system. We will dive more into the frameworks of trauma-informed yoga in Chapter 3, where I will provide more guidance on this concept.

When I look at this visual I ask myself: How can we possibly leave the body out of the equation when it comes to healing from sexual assault? There is an increasing amount of research on the impact of yoga on reducing the symptoms of PTSD. Research supported by the National Institutes of Health shows that 10 weeks of trauma-informed yoga dramatically reduced PTSD symptoms of patients who failed to respond to medication or other types of treatment (West, et al., 2017). You can also see Chapter 2 and visit the appendix to see references to a number of research articles that demonstrate the evidence-based impact of yoga on the healing process for trauma survivors.

## TRAUMA AND THE BRAIN

Having a foundational framework for understanding the impact of trauma on the brain is powerful because it offers practitioners and healing professionals a more holistic scope of the survivor experience. It can also provide more context as to why it might be difficult for a survivor to recall certain details related to their experiences of trauma or to have a linear account of the horror they have experienced. The hope is that it also helps folks infuse more empathy, culturally affirming practices, and compassion into their language, policies, and protocols and reenvision what it truly means to be trauma informed—both as a practitioner and as an agency/institution.

The amygdala is the part of our brain that is responsible for keeping us safe. It is essentially our emotional control center and it is responsible for the fight, flight, and freeze responses. The impact of trauma on the amygdala is that it keeps it in overdrive; survivors may be constantly scanning their environment for danger and imminent threat, even when it may not be present. This is one reason why trauma survivors may constantly live in states of fear, anxiety, or hyperarousal, and why resting and feeling safe can be so difficult (as previously explored).

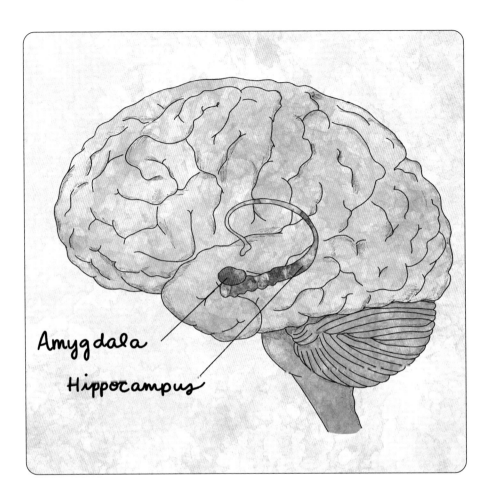

Amygdala

Hippocampus

The hippocampus is the part of our brain that is responsible for the formation of new memories, new concepts, and new skills. And the way these two intersect during trauma is that when the amygdala is constantly searching for threat, the hippocampus gets flooded with a stress hormone known as cortisol. This is what makes it so challenging for survivors to recall certain memories associated with their trauma(s).

A visual I reference in my training, which stems from Rebecca Campbell's (2014) work on the neurobiology of trauma on "the world's messiest desk," is to imagine that you had Post-it Notes all in sequential order on your desk. And someone came over and wiped those Post-its away. Crumpled some. Hid some in drawers. Switched the order of them. Threw others in the trash can. The memories that survivors have associated with their trauma can become incredibly fragmented. And during trauma, the speech center can shut down—making it extremely difficult for survivors to articulate what happened to them in words. Body-based modalities, somatic approaches in therapy, and trauma-informed yoga are a few examples of providing multiple pathways to healing that support safety and stabilization of the nervous system.

We are losing too many survivors who don't feel comfortable coming forward to seek support because sharing details about their experience of trauma is not an accessible or supportive option for them. Many survivors have shared that they have been struggling in isolation, do not have access to other options, or have felt that there were limited resources that were accessible to their needs. Trauma-informed yoga in many ways is creating an avenue for survivors to receive support, feel hope and relief, honor their resilience, and recognize that they are worthy of their own healing and that they don't have to do it alone.

## THE WINDOW OF TOLERANCE

I remember when I used to work at a sexual assault center on a college campus. I loved my job and my work with survivors but I was struggling deeply with my mental health. Every morning before work I would wake up and turn on the news, which meant immediately taking in traumatic stories to begin my day. I would usually check email half asleep in my bed before getting to work—already feeling anxious about my to-do list before I even left my apartment. I would hop in my car and turn on a trauma-related podcast. Once I arrived at work I would be facilitating presentations on trauma, teaching trauma-informed yoga classes, or listening to survivor stories daily. My schedule was back-to-back. I would often eat lunch quickly at my desk, spend time on social media on my breaks (taking in additional trauma headlines), and rarely step outside to see the sun. In case it is not obvious, this type of lifestyle is not recommended! I used to think of caring for myself as something that I did at the end of my day when I had reached the point of emotional and physical exhaustion. Sometimes I would get to my yoga mat at the end of my day and just cry, with nothing left to give my family. My nervous system

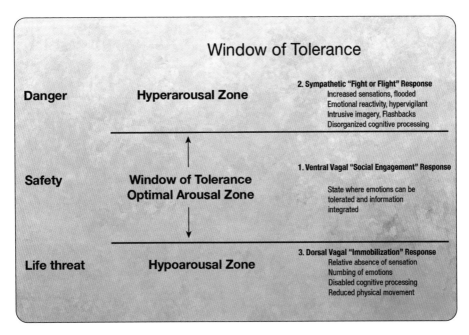

Adapted from "Figure 2.1 Window of Tolerance", from TRAUMA AND THE BODY: A SENSORIMOTOR APPROACH TO PSYCHOTHERAPY by Pat Ogden, Kenkuni Minton, Clare Pain. Copyright © 2006 by Pat Ogden. Copyright © 2006 by W. W. Norton & Company, Inc. Used by permission of W. W. Norton & Company, Inc.

had no space to process anything that felt safe, spacious, or restorative. And all of this compounded with my own unresolved trauma(s) and my lived experience as a woman of color? The perfect recipe for burnout and exhaustion. **Enter: the window of tolerance.**

The "window of tolerance" was a concept developed by Daniel Siegel and is an incredibly informative framework for attuning to the physiological states in the body and creating awareness around when we might be moving in and out of states of dysregulation. It can support us in noticing the practices and habits we are engaging in that are harmful or helpful. One of the quickest alarms for me that I am out of my window of tolerance is that I become incredibly irritable, and I consider myself a pretty compassionate person! My partner usually says something like, "Honey, your empathy meter is in the red." He knows that is one of the quickest ways to communicate to me that I need support or time to return to my practice. Engaging in self- and community care, weaving restorative practices throughout the day, setting boundaries, and constantly evaluating and challenging the systems that create barriers to doing my work in a trauma-informed way have been integral to my survival, energy, bandwidth, capacity, and healing. And now, being a mother, I have found that tools for regulating and tending to my nervous system have never been more important. Anne Lamott shares, "The most profound thing we can offer our children is our own healing." These words have had a big impact on my heart and serve as a constant reminder of the ripple effect of our healing.

Being aware of the physiological signals of my own body allows me to be more intentional with my choices around my time and energy and to create more space to experience ease. Yoga was the first practice that empowered me to be honest with myself, to be aware of my own body, and to name that what I had been experiencing for years was dissociation. I knew that I could not continue down this path. It was not sustainable. The practice created a space for me to approach my well-being in renewed ways. This began with small steps that turned into powerful reframes and rituals.

I don't always get it right, and I stumble and fall back into old patterns that don't serve me, but the healing happens in the moments of acknowledgment and beginning again. I now strive to begin my mornings with a restorative ritual that might include journaling, practicing yoga and meditation, setting intentions, and drinking coffee in the quiet before anyone else wakes up or before checking my phone. I space meetings out and create transitions in my day. I weave self-care practices throughout my day, instead of just at the end. I say no frequently and make it a conscious practice to not fill every minute. I honor the fact that I need a lot more rest than I think I do. I schedule naps and go to therapy (a privilege I know that not every person has access to). I set limits on how often I engage with trauma-related material outside of work. I remind myself that I have hobbies that don't involve trauma! I do fun things with friends. I create intentional and unplugged time with my family and I fiercely protect our time together on weekends. I consistently do something that is incredibly difficult for me: **I ask for help and I am specific about what I need** (which has been its own type of practice). This has been a journey that certainly did not happen overnight. And believe me, unpacking messages related to my own worth is something I have to tend to every day because it has a direct impact on the way I care for myself. But supportive and intentional choices became easier when I started to recognize the distinct and positive impact they had on my mental health. I find that as a trauma survivor, I have to be very intentional about managing my stress, because trauma symptoms can return quickly and with intensity.

Do the very best you can with what you have and where you are in this moment. Start small by taking note of when you are out of your window of tolerance. Make a list of your go-to tools. Start to reevaluate your schedule. You deserve to reclaim your own energy, time, and affection. You are worthy of your own care.

When we are in our window, we feel good. We can perhaps make informed decisions about our needs. We have increased capacity and resources to handle the daily stressors that come our way. Trauma-informed yoga is one modality of many that can support survivors in expanding their window of tolerance and invite them to attend to the accumulation of trauma residue and symptoms they might be carrying in their bodies. It is a tool that can support survivors with their ongoing mental health so they can be mindful of when they may be moving in and out of states of dysregulation and be proactive in how they respond with compassion toward themselves. Sharing this concept in classes or in therapy sessions with survivors can be a powerful and empowering tool for psychoeducation. So let's talk more about how trauma-informed yoga can support the healing process for survivors of sexual assault. Thank you for continuing to journey with me. It means so much that you are here.

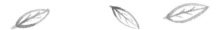

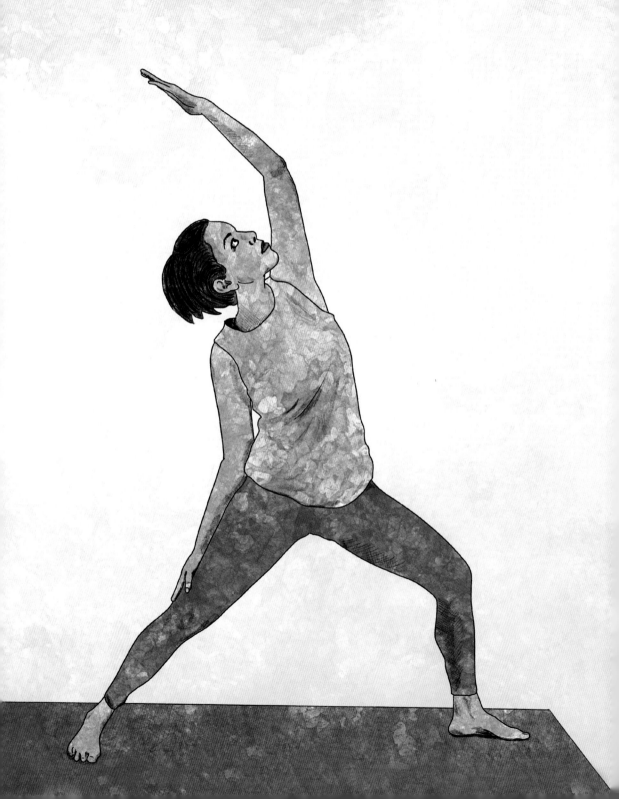

# + 2 +

# How Trauma-Informed Yoga
# Supports Healing

*An embedded trauma response can manifest as fight, flee, or*
*freeze—or as some combination of constriction, pain, fear,*
*dread, anxiety, unpleasant (and/or sometimes pleasant)*
*thoughts, reactive behaviors, or other sensations and*
*experiences. This trauma then gets stuck in the body—*
*and stays stuck there until it is addressed.*
—RESMAA MENAKEM, *MY GRANDMOTHER'S HANDS*

*It is time we think more creatively, more holistically, more*
*honestly and more intentionally about how to best support*
*survivors in healing; move outside of our standard practices*
*and typical referrals to finally meet the body, mind and spiritual*
*needs of our diverse survivor population.*
—MOLLY BOEDER HARRIS, *FOUNDER, THE BREATHE NETWORK*

## Honoring the Lived Experience

*Take some of the radiance you pour out for others and*
*turn it inward to shine on the neglected parts of your soul.*
*It's time.*
—DR.THEMA BRYANT-DAVIS, PHD

**Vinyasa: to place in a special way. In Sanskrit, the term** *nyasa* **means to place and** *vi* **means in a special way.** I remember the first time I really internalized this translation. I remember the joy and space it brought to my practice and the way it transformed the agency of my choices. Those sacred moments in Tadasana (Mountain Pose) where I felt the power of standing in my own truth. Or moving through repeated sun salutations with no other focus than connecting the power of my movement with my breath. Or those times in Virabhadrasana II (Warrior II) or Utthita Tadasana (Star Pose) where I could notice the palpable feeling of taking up space, amid all the ways trauma makes it easy to stay small. And finally the restorative moments in Balasana (Child's Pose) where I spent the entire practice and reminded myself I was worthy of rest. I like to think of my practice as a bridge to my life. The tools I have gained within the four corners of my yoga mat have empowered me to make intentional choices in my healing journey. It was within those four corners that I began to realize I could protect my energy and my peace, and I gradually began to embrace pockets of relief in joy—no matter how fleeting. My practice helped me find words for my feelings and also gave me permission to move forward when words could not do justice. The practice allowed me to feel lighter, more balanced, and grounded. It allowed me to take control of my healing in profound ways.

My practice has shown me what it means to be a steady and safe anchor amid the intense crashing of the waves. The stormy seasons. The trying moments that life inevitably presents in the aftermath of trauma. The practice is always there as a reminder. An integration. A renegotiation. An option to choose another way. A soft place to land. To ground. To feel peace even amid the resistance—even when it's hard.

The practice provides a container for my needs and clarity around what those needs actually are. It offers a compassionate anchor and a place to be held. To release the perfectionism and the need to constantly do. The practice helps me honor my truth. To know, understand, and feel my capacities. To find my own embodied language. It consistently gives me the strength to share my experience authentically—on my own terms and in my own way.

It offers a way to be mindful of my reactions and of what deserves my energy. A place to get lost in the flow of the present. A journey to uncovering the messages behind the trauma imprints that reside inside. It offers a gentle yet powerful reminder of the parts of me that need my own love and my own attention. A place to be reminded that I am inherently whole. A way to return to me. A reminder that I am not defined by my trauma.

Every day I am reminded, as I hold space for survivors through this ancient and sacred practice, that healing from trauma is about honoring our growth (no matter how small that growth feels at times) as well as the nonlinear journey through healing. It is letting ourselves cling to those moments of joy, because we know the deepest pain. There is often no finish line. There is so much to be learned in the mess and in the permission to begin as many times as we need.

Trauma-informed yoga supports survivors in activating their parasympathetic nervous system and creates more space for safety, rest, growth, and abundant joy. When given these tools, survivors can also access greater depths of inner capacity and resilience in navigating not only chronic stress, trauma, and crisis but also the everyday challenges that life presents.

Research has shown that yoga decreases symptoms of hyperarousal, enhances mindfulness, enhances awareness and acceptance of emotions, improves emotion regulation, reduces avoidance and reexperiencing of symptoms, decreases anxiety and depression, and increases resilience (Mitchell et al., 2014). For centuries survivors have also known this to be true in their bodies. Something that has carried me in the process of birthing and writing this book is just how important it is for survivors to be invited to trust in the beauty and power of their own experience.[*]

As a survivor of sexual assault, I never imagined the years of disconnect I would have from my own body without a conscious awareness of what was actually happening. I wasn't prepared for the way my past experiences of trauma would sneak up on me and manifest in various areas of my skin where painful memories were buried and tender. Sometimes, triggers

---

[*] A portion of the following section also appears in *Embodied Resilience Through Yoga*, copyright Llewellyn, 2020.

would create sensations in my limbs, leaving me with a heavy heart and frustration as I sat in anxiousness at the thought of having to explain these physiological symptoms in talk therapy. I carry my most painful and traumatic experiences in my body. The body remembers. Living with trauma can make it really difficult to access parts of ourselves that may feel frozen, numb, or too painful to explore.

In the years that followed the rape in 2007, I felt like shattered pieces of a puzzle. Yoga entered my life at a time when nothing else made sense. In Sanskrit, *yoga* translates to "union." And the practice became integral to helping me recognize that I am inherently whole. It helped me realize that reclaiming choice with my body was going to be an ongoing process for the rest of my life. It gave me the road map to begin the slow journey of putting my pieces back together. I finally had an outlet to process the unsafe feelings that were residing inside of me. Yoga gave me a form of self-expression that allowed me to move beyond the pressure to find the words to articulate what I was feeling. Yoga reminds me each and every day that I am not defined by my experiences of trauma. It has played an instrumental role in the journey of finding a safe home within myself.

**And what I know for sure is that being fully committed to reclaiming my joy is a practice that has held and carried me in my healing.**

## BENEFITS OF TRAUMA-INFORMED YOGA

I knew I wasn't alone in the physiological impact that sexual trauma had on my body. And I felt passionate about connecting with other survivors and supporting them in what can often be an isolating journey. Initially I thought Transcending Sexual Trauma Through Yoga might provide survivors with opportunities to practice self-care and build community. But I have been incredibly moved by the benefits of the practice. We have collected data from thousands of survivors in their healing journey who have participated in the 8-week trauma-informed yoga program across multiple college campuses, and below are some of the ways the practice has shaped and changed their lives and the trajectory of their healing:

- the recognition of choices in one's life
- feelings of safety and strength
- ability to be more expressive in therapy
- positive coping skills, including strengthening inner resources
- self-care strategies
- understanding of how to ask for help
- improved trust in self and others
- development of a strong sense of community
- the establishment of boundaries and understanding of how to be assertive
- the ability to be intimate again
- decreased feelings of depression, stress, and anxiety
- decreased symptoms of PTSD
- empowerment to seek other resources such as counseling, medical support, and/or the gaining of confidence to report the assault to police or Title IX
- increased confidence and courage
- increased feelings of self-compassion
- increased awareness of needs, mindfulness skills, and resiliency
- strengthened self-esteem
- strengthened emotional, physical, mental, spiritual, and inter-personal skills
- increased feelings of being seen, valued, and affirmed

It is important to note that many programs have found that survivors who express a lack of interest in talk therapy have flourished in art- or movement-based formats (Poore et al., 2013). What always remains with me each time I facilitate this program is the capacity of the human spirit to heal amid the unfathomable. When I first meet with a survivor for their intake meeting to discuss their readiness to participate in the trauma-informed yoga program (more on this process in Chapter 5), they share so much about their hopes around healing with me. It is breathtaking to witness their journey from that initial moment and all of the moments that follow as their healing shifts and transcends throughout our 8 weeks together. I can't imagine a greater honor than seeing the tangible impact of the practice and witnessing a survivor's ability to uncover their own resilience.

## A GROWING DEPTH OF RESEARCH AND A CULTURALLY AFFIRMING LENS

There are several studies exploring the impacts of trauma-focused yoga programs on the healing process of participants. **And that really is the critical piece: offering the practice from a trauma-informed lens.** And while the research studies that follow are significant and important contributions to the field, I also want to highlight that so many stories are left out of the mainstream conversation because of the lack of representation of people of color, diverse abilities, and intersecting identities in these spheres. So we always have to hold a critical lens and ask ourselves: Whose stories are not reflected and represented? This is a significant aspect of doing this work from a trauma-informed and intersectional lens. We are committing to the lifelong process of learning and unpacking the specific narratives that are shared. Additionally, it is important to remember that survivors have known and felt the healing impact of ancient and Indigenous practices, like yoga, for centuries—since far before research or funding was possible.

I have always been so moved by the beauty of yogic philosophy, especially Patanjali's eight-limbed path, through the lens of my own healing journey. I spent years in reflection with yogic philosophies and integrated them into my physical, emotional, and spiritual healing journey. When we think about how the practice impacts our lives, it is the greatest reminder that yoga is so much more than just the asana practice. The ripple effect of committing to our healing cannot be measured. I think that as practitioners we cause more harm when we don't honor the roots of the practice. Cultural appropriation is harmful and can cause additional trauma. Before teaching this practice or offering the tools you have learned and will continue to learn, I encourage you to spend time in reflection with the roots and philosophies of the practice. Notice how the tools transform your own life, and make note of the connections to your healing and the healing work you offer. This practice is for everyone and we all have a role in doing this work with integrity and in culturally affirming ways. I encourage you to read Susanna Barkataki's *Embrace Yoga's Roots* to help deepen your practice.

## AN OVERVIEW OF EVIDENCE-BASED RESEARCH ON TRAUMA-INFORMED YOGA

Generally, research has demonstrated that yoga can be an effective intervention to reduce the effects of trauma on mental health (Dick et al., 2014; Emerson et al., 2009; Macy et al., 2018; Mitchell et al., 2014; Rhodes et al., 2016; Telles, 2012). Specifically, an evaluation of a 10-week program indicated that participants noted statistically significant decreases in PTSD symptom severity and greater reductions in depressive symptoms (Rhodes et al., 2016). An evaluation of the Trauma Center Yoga Program revealed that participants demonstrated improvements in all dimensions of PTSD, increases in positive affect, and greater body attunement after 8 weeks of participation in the program (Emerson et al., 2009).

According to Alison Rhodes and colleagues (2016), 10 sessions of yoga helped participants significantly decrease their PTSD symptom severity, decreased experiences of negative tension, and reduced dissociative and depressive symptoms. Trauma-sensitive yoga has been found to be an effective adjunctive and complementary treatment for PTSD (Mitchell et al., 2014). Additionally, there is promise for the incorporation of trauma-sensitive yoga in clinical settings: A study by Cari Jo Clark and colleagues integrated trauma-sensitive yoga into community-based psychotherapy groups for survivors of intimate partner violence. One participant shared, "I didn't have to leave the meeting with anxiety. . . . I was able to leave it on the mat" (Clark et al., 2014).

So what does it actually look like to explore offering survivors of sexual assault the practice of yoga from a trauma-informed lens? That is where we are headed. But first I invite you to take a moment and pause. Perhaps invite some movement into your body that feels nourishing and supportive to you. Take a look back at how far you've come. You are amazing.

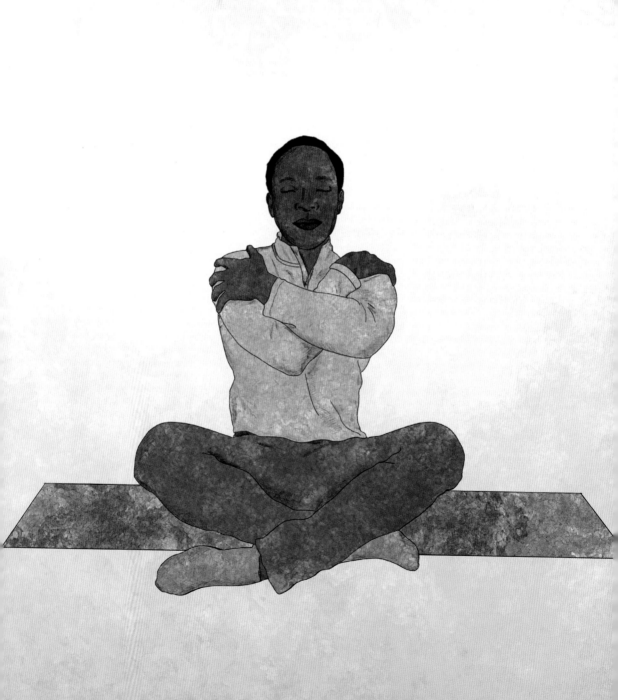

# ✦ 3 ✦

# Teaching Trauma-Informed Yoga

*Can we really continue to leave the body out of the healing process?*
—BO FORBES, *YOGA FOR EMOTIONAL BALANCE*

Ever since I began teaching yoga from a trauma-informed lens, I often take moments to gaze around the room at all of the incredible students who have trusted me with their healing journey. I always say that showing up is the hardest part. I take note of the ways students make intentional choices with their own bodies and step into their strength on their own terms. As I look around the room I notice that no one looks the same and that many students are moving through their own variations of the postures. Some finding rest, others finding movement. I can't help but smile and cherish those moments. It is a beautiful thing to witness survivors feeling safe enough to honor their choices.

Shortly after I was sexually assaulted, I threw myself into graduate school and I focused on sexual assault policy work. And more than anything else: I committed my heart to helping as many survivors as I possibly could. In 2011, I moved through the transformational journey of my 200-hour yoga teacher training and it gave me the space to actually feel. For years I had been frozen and numb. And I was just starting to experience what it felt like to thaw the grief I had been holding internally. For so long my own trauma-healing journey, my sexual assault prevention work on college campuses, and my yoga practice were all very separate, compartmentalized facets of my life. A few years passed before I started recognizing that not only was my yoga practice playing an integral role in my healing, it was also giving me a language to understand the unique, nuanced, and embodied needs of survivors who were sharing their stories with me. I remember one night sitting in my pajamas feeling so incredibly inspired that I wrote out an entire 8-week trauma-informed yoga curriculum. I remember having a blank notebook (which I still have and come back to often) and scribbling down all the ideas that came to mind. My notes included themes that were tailored to the unique experience of survivors, affirmations that grounded them in their own worthiness, journaling prompts that invited them to explore their inner landscape of resilience, sequences that reminded them of their own strength. I was moved by my overarching intention: How can I make this practice accessible to the needs of survivors of sexual assault? The words poured right out of me—honestly, as if they had been waiting to be unlocked for years. It was an incredibly healing form of release. I soon began teaching the series to survivors, and their testimonials moved me beyond words:

> *"I gained my body, spirit, and mind back. I gained confidence, openness, and courage. I gained strength, assertiveness, and knowledge to carry me for a lifetime. I gained myself back."*

> *"This program helped me find my inner voice. Peace. Some courage to be myself and communicate my needs/wants to others. I'm learning how to speak up for myself. This yoga class has changed my life."*

> *"My body is my own and I am the only one who knows how to live in it truthfully."*

> *"I found a way to be calm at my most stressful and emotional times."*

*"Prior to the program, I was having difficulty with eating.
When I would get stressed, either emotionally or with
school, I would have a panic attack and eat until I felt better.
I felt that the satisfaction from eating, as if I was hungry,
calmed me down. I have gained 30 pounds since I was
raped, but I am proud to say that since the beginning of
yoga, I have been able to control my emotions way better
and have stopped eating/binging."*

....................

*"Taking yoga with you gave me hope."*

....................

*"I learned that being who I am is enough."*

In 2012 I attended a 40-hour training on trauma-sensitive yoga led by Jenn Turner, David Emerson, and Bessel van der Kolk. It validated so many of my insights into the practice, inspired me, and provided me with a language and foundation to build upon in my work with survivors of sexual assault. And now, 8 years later, there is so much I have experienced through my own lens of trauma, and the realization of the unique pieces around the cultural implications of the practice. As a woman of color, as a survivor of sexual assault, birth trauma, and the loss of a child, and having supported my mother and husband through their own unique cancer journeys, I have experienced profound shifts in the way I hold space for myself and others through a trauma-informed lens. And that curriculum I told you about that I wrote in the wee hours of the morning? I never imagined in a million years that it would be implemented at over 30 universities and trauma agencies across the country. Something I have learned that feels important to share: **Trust the power of your voice and the anchor of your own truth.**

As mentioned earlier, teaching from a trauma-informed lens is a lifelong process that evolves over time through our learning and is informed by the lived experiences of all those we hold space for. It is an ongoing commitment, a philosophy, and an (ever-evolving) systemic framework of the way we truly see people and honor their humanity. It is a persistent and dedicated commitment to being an ally, staying informed and educating ourselves, practicing humility, and engaging in inclusive and affirming practices. A good starting point is to think about the tenets of trauma-informed care and apply them to the way we hold space for survivors. This chapter will review the following frameworks for those who are interested in teaching trauma-informed yoga to survivors of sexual assault and/or integrating these concepts into the scope of your work or healing: (1) empowerment-based language, (2) supportive presence and the embodied practice of holding space, (3) self- and community care for the teacher, (4) consent and physical assists in yoga spaces, (5) creating safety in the physical yoga space, (6) a trauma-sensitive approach to breath work and mindfulness, (7) supporting students who are triggered, and (8) cultural considerations and accessibility. **Please note that the frameworks are taught from a broad lens and the concepts can be applied to working with multiple populations of trauma across many different professions.**

## 1. Empowerment-Based Language

Survivors of sexual assault have lost so much power and control over their own bodies. I believe the use of empowering, compassionate, supportive, and invitational language is the core component of teaching yoga to survivors to give them a sense of control over their own lives. We are using our language as a means of creating transformation. Of grounding students in their own worthiness. Of reminding them that they are enough just as they are and that the intentional choices they make with their own bodies are celebrated. It is the difference between giving a direct instruction versus offering the experience to go inward and explore their own internal landscape and sense of embodied safety. We are supporting survivors as they navigate and trust the intelligence of their own bodies. Our language absolutely matters.

In many ways the practice of yoga has become westernized and culturally appropriated, and so has the normalization of "push harder, sit deeper" language. Our lives are hard enough—our practice doesn't have to be. What ends up happening is we begin replicating the busyness, the pushing, and the overworking as a parallel process on our mat. This is also a greater analogy for so many aspects of our lives. Bo Forbes (2011) shares, "Our cultural conditioning toward big changes and instant results can cause many of us to overlook the power of these subtle practices." The healing can happen in the compassionate awareness of these slow, intentional moments over time. Survivors deserve to explore the softness of their practice and to receive embodied messages around celebrating rest. This is the first step toward inspiring daily practices that help activate the parasympathetic nervous system.

If you have ever taken a yoga class before, think about how many times you have heard an instructor say, "Everybody needs a strap and two blocks." When we teach from a trauma-informed lens, this statement might look like, "I will be inviting the use of props into our practice today. If it feels comfortable for you, please feel free to use a strap and two blocks." What do you notice within your own body when you sense the shift between these statements? When we invite choice and make even subtle shifts in our language, it can help to bring ease to a survivor's nervous system. Here are a few other examples of what this might look like in practice:

**Instead of:**
"Stay in the room the entire time and drink water only at the designated breaks."

**Perhaps try:**
"You are welcome to leave the room at any time and drink water as you need. Your comfort and safety are the most important elements of your practice."

**Instead of:**
"Lie on your back and be still."

**Perhaps try:**
"You are worthy and welcome to explore what savasana looks like in your body. You could explore multiple variations of rest. Know that you can move or shift at any time to increase your sense of safety."

**Instead of:**

"Close your eyes."

**Perhaps try:**

"You can keep your eyes open, find a soft gaze, or close them if that feels comfortable for you."

Below are sample trauma-informed cues, affirmations, and phrases you might consider integrating into your work with survivors or to support your own healing. Feel free to spend some time here. Circle the ones that resonate with you. Have your journal handy in case you feel inspired to write your own. Notice how the language lands on your own heart. For the survivors who are reading this section, you might even integrate the compassionate phrases and affirmations into your own daily ritual, journaling practice, or intention setting.

### Sample Trauma-Informed Cues

- *The choices you make with your body are always celebrated here.*
- *You are always in control of your practice.*
- *You are your greatest teacher.*
- *I invite you to send yourself gratitude just for arriving to your mat today. So often that is the hardest part.*
- *I invite you to take a moment to reflect on your journey and how far you've come. Inhale and exhale at your pace.*
- *Today explore taking up all the space you deserve.*
- *Know that you are welcome to leave at any time. Your comfort and safety are the most important elements of your practice.*
- *All of you is welcome here.*
- *You are worthy of choice.*
- *You are enough, exactly as you are.*
- *You have many options to explore what rest looks like for you.*
- *There are many ways to communicate your comfort level with assists. I honor your choices and you can change your mind at any time.*

- *If being with the internal sensations feels too overwhelming, know that you can explore focusing on something external in the room, outside of your body. Perhaps a color, sound, scent—choose what feels soothing and supports you in reorienting to the space.*
- *Feel free to modify the posture to increase your comfort. You can come out of the posture at any time.*
- *Know that you can keep your eyes open, close them, or find a soft gaze. This is your body and always your choice.*
- *Allow being where you are to be enough. It is enough.*
- *I invite you to explore finding a shape in your body that feels safe and supportive to you.*

**Compassionate Phrases to Help Ease a Survivor's Nervous System**

- *There is no rush.*
- *Take all the time you need.*
- *Your resilience inspires me.*
- *I'm here to support you in whatever way feels best for you.*
- *It's your choice. I support you with my whole heart.*
- *Thank you for trusting me.*
- *It's okay to feel exactly what you feel. I'm here holding the hope with you.*
- *How is your heart?*
- *I see the light in you.*
- *Your journey is brave.*
- *I see your courage. You have come so far.*
- *It's okay to rest and go slow.*
- *I see you.*
- *You are not alone in this experience.*
- *I believe you.*
- *Your needs matter.*
- *What happened to you is not your fault.*
- *You are worthy of gentleness, kindness, and peace.*
- *Healing is possible. In your way, at your pace.*
- *May you trust in the beauty of your individual journey.*

**Survivor Affirmations**

- *I am not alone in this experience.*
- *I deserve to take up space.*
- *I honor the layers of my unique lived experience.*
- *My light shines even in the dark.*
- *I honor the layers and intersections of my unique lived experience.*
- *I am healing, even when it's hard.*
- *I acknowledge the challenges with caring for myself, but I try anyway.*
- *I trust the strength of my body to hold me today.*
- *I am worthy of rest.*
- *I will not doubt my value and my power.*
- *I deserve to live with ease.*
- *I am not my trauma.*
- *I am safe. I am loved. I am home. I am in my body.*
- *My healing is not linear, and that is okay.*
- *I remember it is okay to ask for help and receive support.*
- *There is beauty in my emotions.*
- *I am allowed to protect my energy.*
- *I honor the waves of healing.*
- *I will not shrink.*
- *I am brave.*
- *I am showing up exactly as I am.*
- *I am listening to my body.*
- *I deserve peace.*
- *My needs are important.*
- *I honor my boundaries.*
- *I am learning to love me.*
- *What happened to me was not my fault.*
- *I am not defined by how much I do.*
- *I trust my gifts.*
- *I release shame. It does not belong here with my heart.*
- *I am held and supported.*

- *I am creating space for joy.*
- *I deserve larger margins in my day and space between things.*
- *I am resilient.*

As you might have noticed, every cue is an invitation. I first learned about invitational language in my training with the Justice Resource Institute and I have witnessed a profound shift in the comfort it creates for survivors in their practice. The phrases above come straight from my heart and from the years I have spent holding space for survivors. Paying attention to their precious words and the experiences they have bravely shared with me. Noticing the softening that happens when words affirm their existence and their needs. I think there is something powerful about the energy and community that are shared between survivors. The connection and healing are felt in the physicality of the space. They create a sense of community that transcends words.

As you become more acquainted with your own authentic teaching voice and with language that feels comfortable for you, I want to invite you to consider using transition words between each of the postures to affirm and validate the reminders and choices that survivors have with their bodies. Offer them the flexibility to explore their body on their own terms. Release the ego and the dynamic involved with the hierarchy of teacher and student. You might find yourself feeling self-conscious by how often you are using invitations. But I promise you: **You cannot remind survivors enough about the choices they have with their own bodies**.

And just as there are different styles of psychotherapy, and the fit between a survivor and therapist is so important, there are also different styles of yoga. And contrary to what might be expected, this type of language can actually be integrated into any type of practice you might be offering. To give you some context, one of the first places I started teaching yoga from a trauma-informed lens was actually at a CrossFit gym. CrossFit is a very physically challenging practice and I would often lead a class in the evenings after participants' workouts. It was quite moving to see the students invite in softness and come into their bodies in a completely different way, often through the subtle and supportive shifts in the language I was sharing. Eventually this became more intuitive and embodied for them and it was beautiful to witness them honor their innate body wisdom *on their own*. So much of the practice is inviting students to listen to their bodies and respond in ways that feel kind and compassionate.

If you are a therapist who is exploring integrating this language and practice into your clinical practice, you might explore saying something from Amy Weintraub, author of *Yoga Skills for Therapists*: "Would you like to try a new approach to help calm that revved up feeling you are experiencing?" (Linda Crossley, personal communication, June 2014). Trauma-informed embodied practices can provide a supportive gateway to processing trauma narratives. These restorative practices invite survivors to have space to arrive, find some semblance of stabilization and safety in their nervous system, and invite them to gently reacquaint themselves with their own breath. There are so many small ways to explore integrating trauma-informed yoga into your clinical practice (e.g., centering practice, setting an intention followed by brief meditation before verbal processing, seated sun salutations, grounding practices, safe visualizations). This will be further explored in Chapter 5.

If you are an educator or facilitator, you might consider beginning your classes, lectures, trainings, or workshops with seated sun salutations, a grounding practice, or exploring with trauma-informed breath options. When I facilitate presentations on trauma, I am acutely aware of the elements of my presentations that might be triggering. Taking a few moments to integrate trauma-informed yoga at both the beginning and end of my lectures allows me to honor the fact that folks show up in these spaces with their full mind, body, and spirit. The information they are learning is going to impact them and land in different ways based on their lived experience. By intentionally integrating embodiment into our spaces of learning, we can empower students to honor what their bodies are communicating to them when we are working with difficult, heavy, and challenging topics. I recall so many times during my undergraduate and graduate career where I forced myself to sit in lectures and learn about material that completely overwhelmed my nervous system. I rarely had the option to safely integrate what I was learning, opt out, or honor the full senses of my body as it related to material I was absorbing. These small steps to integrate these practices into the various facets of our lives can create a compassionate place to land amid the many ways trauma surrounds our world and our experiences.

So whether you are a fitness instructor, a yoga teacher, a therapist, a social-justice educator, a survivor advocate, a doula, a medical professional, a faculty member or student affairs professional, a friend or family member of a survivor, or someone who is passionate about working with survivors of sexual assault—begin with your words. Explore integrating the softness of this language into the scope of your work and interactions. And start to take note of the profound shifts that happen in helping survivors feel seen and cared for.

## A NOTE ON PRESCRIPTIVE CUES WHEN WORKING WITH SURVIVORS

I want to invite you to be cognizant of saying statements like "This posture is very good for relieving anxiety or depression" or "This is how to get into the full expression of the posture." All bodies are unique and there is no one-size-fits-all approach when it comes to healing from sexual assault. We cannot assume that folks in our classes or spaces are going to be having the same experience. The beauty of the practice is that students get to decide what feels most supportive to them. Teaching from a trauma-informed lens is less about specific asanas (sequences or postures) and more about the empowering invitation for students to access safety and embodiment. Additionally, in a variety of mindfulness practices, you may hear the statement, "Send love and light to people who have hurt you." Hearing this statement in the context of contemplative practice can be incredibly triggering for a survivor and is a concept known as spiritual bypassing. Spiritual bypassing is a way of dishonoring the real feelings and emotions that students may be experiencing by providing blanket or overarching statements around spirituality or enlightenment. A survivor does not owe their perpetrator forgiveness. A statement like this can actually exacerbate their symptoms of traumatic stress.

Additionally, you might consider avoiding cueing postures or saying phrases that could be triggering specifically to survivors of sexual assault, which might include Halasana (Plow Pose), Ananda Balasana (Happy Baby), and anything exposing the pelvic area. Words you might consider avoiding include "Corpse Pose," "knife edge of the foot," and "grind." If you are teaching classes specifically to survivors, I invite you to share general supportive statements to affirm the experience of every single person in the room and not single people out. An example of this might be, "Beautiful expressions, everyone. I love the ways each of you are honoring choices with your bodies today." Highlighting or affirming the choices that survivors make only when they are in the most advanced form of the posture adds to the daily messages that we should be "pushing harder" or "doing more." We receive these messages constantly in the context of our sympathetic dominant (i.e., stressful) world. Our language is a powerful tool that we can offer when teaching yoga, to affirm that rest is one of the most productive choices we can make for ourselves. When we shift our language in this way, we can also help expand the capacity that survivors have to explore and internalize what rest means both on and off their mats.

## 2. Supportive Presence and the Embodied Practice of Holding Space

*Being heard feels like rest.*
—VYANA NOVUS

The best way I can describe this framework is the way you authentically step into the space every time you teach. As shared in the previous chapter, in the context of trauma recovery, until the stress-response system within our bodies is functioning well and has flow and space, it can be incredibly challenging to access safety. Until we feel safe, there may be barriers to accessing vasanas (emotional/residual imprints) that live in the body as a result of traumatic experiences. When we are in crisis or experiencing a trauma trigger, our autonomic nervous system shuts down the activity of the ventral branch of the vagus nerve (Rosenberg, 2017). Trauma symptoms (reference examples in Chapter 1) can lead to a survivor having poor vagal tone, which is the activity of the vagus nerve. The vagus nerve is fundamental to the functioning of the parasympathetic branch of the autonomic nervous system and to emotional regulation. Something important to keep in mind is that in addition to the actual practice of trauma-informed yoga, our safe and supportive presence can also help a survivor engage positively with the ventral branch of their vagus nerve. This creates the capacity for survivors to experience rest in a way that feels accessible. Having a supportive presence allows survivors to experience a safe connection and attunement to another human being. This creates a container where people can begin to heal.

## BOUNDARIES

As with everything we have discussed so far, the elements of safety, trust, choice, and control are critical. This entails maintaining appropriate boundaries and doing so from a trauma-informed lens. A few years ago I read this quote by Yvette Lalonde: "When someone demonstrates healthy boundaries to me, I find that I feel safer in their presence" (Yvette Lalonde, @innerflow_wellness, Instagram, November 1, 2018). I found myself reading it over and over again and thinking about the gift of living in a world where boundaries are supported, affirmed, and encouraged. Where assertive and compassionate communication is embedded into our social constructs. In the context of your role as a healing professional, I want to invite you to think about what it looks like to foster a supportive space while also setting limits with kindness. Additionally, depending on the various intersecting identities that a survivor may hold, their relationship to boundaries may look different, nuanced, and complex. This is important to remember, as it informs how we might speak about boundaries in a way that honors the many layers of someone's unique lived experience and trauma history.

When you begin offering this practice, you may find that survivors feel comfortable disclosing their story to you and/or perhaps sharing details about their experience. You have done an amazing job creating a supportive container if a survivor feels safe to share their experience with you. There are so many ways you can affirm their experience, but always be mindful of what is and what is not within your scope of practice. You can be a supportive and grounding presence for a survivor, while also connecting them to a variety of different resources that call for different kinds of professional expertise and experience (ex: support groups, sliding scale therapists, online options, healing resources, written resources, community referrals, hotline numbers to access confidential support) to support them in verbally processing their trauma(s). It is important to ensure that participants have a clear understanding of the goals and objectives of the trauma-informed yoga program and are clear that it is not clinical therapy or a support group. This helps to ensure that you are staying within your scope of practice and the survivors you are holding space for are getting the appropriate care they need. Here is an example of a way I have communicated this:

> *Thank you so much for trusting me with your story and sharing your experience with me. I imagine that being in this yoga class brings up so many feelings and emotions and I want to ensure I am connecting you to additional resources in your healing journey. I am here to support and empower you in reconnecting to your body in a way that feels supportive and accessible to you. I wanted to share some referrals with you of professionals who are trained to speak with you about what you are going through. You are always in choice about what feels best for you, but I wanted you to have this information in case you may find it supportive. Your courage inspires me. It means so much to hold space for you and connect you to additional care that feels right for you.*

## LISTENING TO FEEDBACK AND MAKING CHANGES

In many instances, those survivors who want to set boundaries and assert their needs the most may struggle to communicate them. Creating an easeful way for survivors to share feedback with you about their experience in your class can help to ensure their needs are being met. Affirming, honoring, and validating people's feelings is one of the most important aspects of our work as practitioners. This allows us to communicate, "I see you. Your needs matter. Thank you so much for telling me how I can make this experience better for you." How people feel is real. This is not a time to get defensive. Take time to process. Be compassionate with yourself and your humanness. Have a system of support in place as you do this work. Honor the courage it takes for someone to communicate their needs and follow up by taking the time to make the changes in your classes and check in with the student. This could be anything from the setup or temperature in the room to the music played, the pace of the class, the language, and the use of candles, among many other elements. We will discuss more about creating safety in the physical space later in this chapter.

## WORKING WITH SURVIVORS OF MARGINALIZED IDENTITIES

Survivors of sexual assault hold many intersecting identities that inform their experience of trauma and healing. These identities must be deeply held and understood because as shared previously, trauma-informed care is not complete without also holding an anti-oppression and intersectional lens. Women of color, queer and trans students, and students with disabilities experience even higher rates of sexual violence compared to their counterparts (Harris et al., 2017; Testa & Dermen, 1999). There are already so many barriers in place for folks in larger bodies, people of color, people in differently abled bodies, LGBTQ folks, people of every race and socioeconomic status, non-binary and gender-nonconforming folks, and those who hold marginalized identities—preventing them from practicing yoga in an accessible way. This can include but is certainly not limited to the financial accessibility of classes, ableism, misogyny and/or sexism, racism, homophobia, transphobia, cultural appropriation of yoga practices, geographic location, and the physical accessibility of the space.

Having a supportive presence involves the deep and committed work of allyship. It is a lifelong commitment to holding space in a way that ensures all survivors feel seen and supported. This doesn't mean we are going to get it right all the time. Healing professionals may fear they will say the wrong thing and as a result make those who hold marginalized identities feel invisible. As shared previously, navigating life after experiencing sexual assault can already feel like an invisible pain. And the added layers of holding multiple intersecting identities, compounded by the trauma of sexual assault and systemic racism, can make this experience unbearable. Survivors deserve support that honors all parts of their humanity. It is an integral piece of our work and must be integrated into all aspects of how we hold space. We will explore some tangible ways to do this later in the chapter.

## CONSISTENCY AND REPETITION AND THEIR ROLE IN SUPPORTING A DYSREGULATED NERVOUS SYSTEM

When working with trauma-informed yoga teachers, I often remind them that it is okay to take the pressure off themselves to create fancy flows or sequences. Consistency and repetition can play a critical role in supporting a survivor who may be struggling with a dysregulated nervous system. When I teach trauma-informed yoga, we may begin with some grounding postures, make our way up through a few sun salutations and warrior postures, and then make our way back down to the mat. So many survivors have shared how they appreciate knowing what to expect each week and how it has played a central role in helping them access safety and develop trust with the teacher. One survivor shared how much they appreciated the consistency of the day and time of class each week because it helped them get in the routine of dedicating specific time to their own healing. They specifically shared, *"I look forward to yoga on Tuesday nights. I used to have a hard time looking forward to any day ahead."*

## CREATING MULTIPLE LAYERS

*I'm learning to feel safe inside my own body. Breathing and making conscious decisions has helped me take my power back. I can choose to stay in a comfortable place or I can choose to stretch myself as far as I choose to. . . . The most important thing here is that I have a choice. I have choices. I am no longer trapped or tied down by my past. It is now a daily choice to lift my head and keep going on this path of light. I may fall off track for a moment but lately it has been easier to remember that I am still on the path of goodness. I no longer say, "I am here but I'm a survivor." I say, I am a survivor and I am here.*

*—EVE ANDRY*

This is a moving testimonial from Eve, who found agency and power in her choices not just on the mat but in her life. An important aspect of teaching from a trauma-informed lens is not only using empowering and choice-based language but also offering multiple variations within each posture. This invites survivors to explore options and honor their bodies when they need something different, and it also gives them the space to challenge themselves when they feel ready to do so. It is a supportive inquiry and an invitation for survivors to come into their own bodies, on their own terms. There are times when I may invite survivors to explore Cobra Pose and on a particular day they may feel ready to move through a Chaturanga. Watching them make small choices, build their strength, and integrate incremental changes in their practice is beautiful to witness, and it often parallels the overall healing process.

## ORIENT STUDENTS TO THE SPACE

It is important to take time to orient survivors to the space as they arrive, at the beginning of class, and throughout your time together. As we have discussed, dissociation is a common experience for survivors. Before jumping right into the practice, I invite you to take precious time to create a space where students can tend to and settle their nervous systems and find comfort in the physical space. A few things to consider:

> ■ Welcome students into the space as they arrive (think back to the elements of supportive presence) and invite them to find a space in the room to set up that feels comfortable to them. Remind them they can set up anywhere in the room that feels right, utilize any of the props available in the space, or share with you directly about ways you can help increase their comfort in the space. I would also recommend making this a frequent practice to reiterate the power and control they have in creating their own space. **You cannot remind survivors enough of the choices they have with their own bodies.**
>
> *(list continued on next page)*

*(list continued from previous page)*

- Explain the consent-affirming protocols around physical assists.
- Explain where they can access gender-neutral restrooms.
- Let them know they are welcome to leave at any time or do anything to increase their comfort during class.
- Take time to set ground rules or community agreements or inform students what existing ones look like and how they can add to them.
- Invite students to identify an inner resource, intention, mantra, or another grounding exercise that they can connect with before class begins. This can support them in accessing a tool in case they feel triggered during the practice.

## SHOWING UP IS THE HARDEST PART

One of the first things I say when students arrive to class is, "Take a few moments to connect with the fact that you made it to your mat today. So often that is the hardest part. Please know that if you wanted to find one shape of rest that really resonates with you and stay there for the next hour— that would be perfect and supported. I honor you just for being here today." When I take note of the way these words land for students in class, I can see and feel an immediate sense of relief in their bodies. I try to remind survivors often that rest is a radical practice and that there are so many ways to explore what that means for them. Inviting in moments of abundant ease and creating opportunities for survivors to be reminded that rest is celebrated, especially for those who may live in constant states of hyperarousal or struggle with the ongoing impact of trauma symptoms and PTSD—this is a beautiful gift.

Your presence alone can create the environment where nonjudgment is felt in the room. One of my favorite quotes by Maya Angelou is "Your energy introduces you before you even speak." I have it written in all of my journals that hold inspiration, quotes, and sequences for my yoga classes. It serves as an anchor for me in doing trauma-informed work with integrity. It reminds me how integral my own practice is to holding a strong container when I teach. Trauma-informed frameworks hold the deep know-ing that teachers and practitioners are our greatest resource. Engaging in regular practices and rituals to support your own mental health is one of the most important ways to do this work in ongoing and sustainable ways. And that is exactly where we are headed and what we will unpack together.

## 3. Self- and Community Care for the Teacher

*A question to ask yourself often: How does this person, space, job, etc. support the health of my nervous system? Explore listening for the answers with the full senses of your mind, body and spirit. You deserve to be intentional and discerning with your energy.*

*I am deeply empathic. Therefore I rest.*
—DR. JAIYA JOHN, *FREEDOM:*
   *MEDICINE WORDS FOR YOUR BRAVE REVOLUTION*

I want to invite you to think back to the concept of the window of tolerance. What are some of the first signs that indicate to you that you are outside of your window? Maybe take a moment to pause here and journal what comes up for you. According to Bo Forbes, "the more empathic we are, the more vulnerable we are to both emotional and sensory contagion, to experiencing someone's emotions and sensations as though they were our own" (personal communication, December 10, 2016). This can impact us at the most visceral level, including manifesting as some of the trauma symptoms mentioned in Chapter 1. Committing to teaching survivors is the most profound and rewarding decision that I have ever made in my career. However, without the appropriate support, supervision, boundar-ies, personal practices, and commitment to self- and community care, it can lead to feelings of exhaustion, compassion fatigue, vicarious trauma, and/or burnout. There are two inquiries I have learned over the years from Dr. Shena Young and Nicole Steward that have made a profound impact on the way I honor my own capacity and hold space. "Are you absorbing, or observing?" (Shena Young, personal communication, April 6, 2018). "Are you carrying, or caring?" (Nicole Steward, personal communication, July 11, 2018). I want to invite you to take an inhale in at your pace, and exhale out in your way. What comes up for you as you think about these inquiries in the scope of your work? And if you tend to absorb and carry, what practices can you weave throughout your day to create more space, ease, and help you reclaim time for yourself? For me, this is about acknowledging the practices that are integral to our overall mental health and long-term well-being.*

I will be honest. It is really challenging for me to rest. To truly rest. I've always been acutely aware that overworking is one of my coping strategies. When responsibilities feel endless, it can feel impossible to find ways to release the tendency to constantly "do" and be in motion. It takes care and intentionality to be present with what is in front of me. To turn down the mental chatter and the urgency of the needs of others. To release the guilt that comes with saying no. Some days the anxiety feels like the most overwhelming visceral emotion that swirls around in my gut. It takes over. As if my nervous system has completely collapsed. And it leads to feelings of depletion.

Self-care for me is an everyday practice that entails attuning to my internal states and resources with discernment. It is about taking embodiment breaks. Creating transitions in my workday. Taking a mindful approach to my relationships and identifying the ones that no longer serve me. It is engaging in activities that nourish and support my nervous system. It is honoring my boundaries and my capacity in ongoing ways. It is being mindful of the harmful systems that impact my well-being and that are out of my control. When we can be gentle and give ourselves permission to ask for what we need, it can be our most powerful resource in recovery. I have learned that caring for myself and asking for help also ensures that those I love and hold space for can also thrive. I remind myself often that I don't have to do it all. When I take on what is within my capacity alone

---

* A portion of the following section also appears in *Embodied Resilience Through Yoga*, copyright Llewellyn, 2020.

and practice self-compassion, I can do my work in ways that feel energizing, restorative, and most importantly—sustainable. Jane Clapp, Jungian Analyst in training and somatic coach, shares a powerful question that can support us with honoring our own capacity in ongoing ways: "Before we take on more commitments, we might consider asking our bodies for consent" (personal communication, 2020). We deserve to normalize statements such as: I can't take that on; I am at capacity with my workload; I can't prioritize that at the moment; I appreciate you thinking of me, but I can't add anything else at this time; No. Your energy is precious and you are worthy of protecting it.

A practice that grounds me is taking the time to remember what my anchors are and what my WHY is. A few years ago I was teaching a weekly trauma-informed yoga class at a donation-based yoga studio in the community. There was a woman in her 60s who traveled an hour and a half to take class with me every single week. I knew that if she was doing the hard work to show up for herself, I would also commit to the same. Sometimes that meant being intentional with giving myself adequate transition time before I was going to lead class. Other times it was taking 10 minutes to meditate in my car if I was short on time. There are so many subtle restorative practices we can weave in and integrate throughout the course of our day to support us with expanding our window of tolerance. This awareness and practice alone can be a tremendous gift to ourselves and help us have more bandwidth and capacity to hold space for others.

And what I know for sure is that the first step to reinforcing our self-worth on a daily basis is recognizing each day that we are worthy of our own love. Like anything else, it is a practice, and not a linear one. It takes all that we have to continue coming back to ourselves, to reevaluate our current practices and identify what needs to change, where we need to recalibrate our boundaries, and when we need to ask for help. It is digging deep and listening to the internal voice that holds so much wisdom. We just have to listen.

I want to make it clear that this is about so much more than self-care. This is about examining the systems of oppression that make it challenging for healing professionals to thrive. No matter how many coping tools we have, we deserve to work for organizations that are truly trauma informed and hold the needs of their staff with integrity, compassion, equity, and action. Educators, therapists, mental health professionals, social workers, and trauma and healing professionals are consistently holding space for others in a myriad of ways amid so much collective trauma. I continue to see so many BIPOC colleagues being tapped for more work when they are already beyond their capacity and asked to give more. There has been little reprieve, and as someone who is witness to some of the most incredible resilience, I keep asking myself how much more people can hold. Sonya Passi, founder of FreeFrom, an organization "whose mission is to dismantle the nexus between intimate partner violence and financial insecurity," shares, "Investing in the people that work in social justice—paying them well, honoring their downtime, and supporting them with good benefits—is the only way we have a chance at building sustainable change" (FreeFrom, @freefromdotorg, Instagram, December 18, 2019). We need systems that prioritize our well-being, mental health, and value—more than ever. We need more than appreciation; we need flexibility, change, resources, and tangible, holistic support—and a reflection of that in the systems that are supposed to care for us. This is more than offering compassion-fatigue trainings. This is an ongoing process that must be approached from multiple angles and systems of care. Institutions, trauma agencies, and mental health centers must frequently revisit and recalibrate their plans and policies to prioritize the well-being of their staff. They must be willing to take an honest look at the systemic conditions and culture that is harming the mental health of their staff. Reminder: **Your mental health always matters.**

Below are a few questions, supportive tools, invitations, embodied inquiries, and rituals related to managing stress, anxiety, and trauma symptoms. These may be of use to you, or you can share them with your students or clients. I invite you to have your journal nearby and take time to develop a unique plan that is tailored to your specific needs and lived experience.

- Reflection questions:
  - *What do I need more or less of?*
  - *Who can I go to for support?*

- *What does this moment require of me?*
- *How can I be challenged but not overcome?*
- *What risks do I need to take to reclaim my joy?*
- *What brings me a sense of well-being and ease?*
- *What systems of oppression are in place that challenge my sense of well-being? Where am I unfairly blaming myself?*

- Check in with your tendency to fill free time on your calendar. Can you reclaim that time for you instead?
- What boundaries need to be explored or communicated, and to whom?
- Are you getting proper supervision, mentorship, and support to manage your current workload? How can you access the support you need to ensure you are not doing this work in isolation? What policy changes can be made to support your well-being? What type of advocacy needs to happen by those in senior leadership positions?
- Explore implementing morning and evening rituals to begin and end your day in supportive, empowering, peaceful, and restorative ways.
- Could you wake up a little earlier to do a short yoga practice, journaling, and intention setting? Or perhaps have some time alone instead of checking email or social media, which can activate your nervous system before you are fully awake.
- Try to limit trauma intake and avoid constant stimulation (phone, screens, overscheduling).
- Journal affirmations and mantras that you can return to during stressful moments.
- Can you give yourself multiple breaks or adequate space between meetings, appointments, and so on, to avoid rushing? If that is not possible, can you practice finding mindful moments amid the chaos to find resource?
- Try to have walking meetings or spend time in nature to recharge and create space for when you may be experiencing stress.

- Can you take mental health days or explore working remotely during times when you feel overwhelmed?
- Can you explore listening to something uplifting or restorative when driving or walking?
- Perhaps try batching your email to avoid constant checking, or have designated phone-free time.
- Ask and receive help. Practice self-compassion.
- Can you plan ahead and give yourself space to have larger margins in your day for more ease?
- What would sacred rituals for a good night's sleep look like for you (e.g., essential oils, eye-mask pillow, tea, baths, Yoga Nidra, breathing practices, stretching)?
- Have or explore routines to stabilize your nervous system.
- Can you drink water, stay nourished throughout the day, and spend time on Sundays to meal-plan for the week?
- If possible and if it feels supportive, schedule consistent therapy appointments.
- Practice presence.
- Schedule time with friends. Lean into your community.
- Can you explore giving less of yourself away at work so you have more time for you and your family?
- What would it look like to give yourself the space and time you need to respond instead of react?
- If you notice resentment or burnout building and arising in your body, can you get curious about the root cause and ask yourself: What does this moment require?
- It's exhausting to feel like you always have to be "on." Are there areas where you can cut back or delegate or where someone else can take the lead?
- Check in with your inner landscape. Throughout the day can you check in with what your body is communicating to you? How might you respond in ways that feel kind and compassionate? Deep breaths. Be gentle with you and your experience.

- Explore with portioning, a somatic tool I learned from my dear colleague Jo Buick. This tool empowers you to be intentional about managing your energy. Take time to assess your energy levels each week (full capacity vs. fatigued), adjust your schedule and expectations of yourself accordingly, and schedule restorative time especially during weeks when you feel depleted (Jo Buick, @jo.buick, Instagram, April 21, 2021).
- Practice self-compassion mantras. One I come back to often is from Dr. Susana M. Muñoz: "I'm not behind or unproductive. I'm doing as much as my mind and body are allowing me to do under perpetual stress and fatigue" (@SusanaPhD, Twitter, October 4, 2020).

## 4. Consent and Physical Assists in Yoga Spaces

*I'm not interested in spending time in any movement or healing space that does not vehemently commit to creating a consent culture.*
—JANE CLAPP, *JUNGIAN ANALYST IN TRAINING AND SOMATIC COACH*

There is so much to say and an incredible amount of nuance involved regarding the intersection of consent, touch, and trauma in yoga spaces. Please know that opinions on this may shift depending on some of the following: folks who are teaching closed trauma-informed yoga classes to survivors; those who might be integrating trauma-informed frameworks into existing classes; and/or therapists, healing professionals, or educators who are integrating this modality into the scope of their work. The one common denominator? **Consent**.

We must be mindful of creating consent frameworks and structures of safety in yoga studios and spaces when it comes to offering physical assists. It is hard to reconcile that in so many movement spaces, the assumption is that it is okay to touch people. Students are often asked to opt out of being touched. Yet the burden should never be placed on students to communicate this. Below I have outlined a number of considerations and recommendations related to assists in the context of yoga.

**Factors to Consider:**

- The Trauma Center at the Justice Resource Institute sees physical assists as a clinical issue and instead they recommend only verbal cues.
- It can be extremely triggering for survivors to be touched without their permission.
- I invite you to consider the implications of dissociation, shared previously. Dissociation is one of the many "defense mechanisms the brain can use to cope with the trauma of sexual violence." It's often described as an "out of body" experience where someone feels detached from reality (RAINN, n.d.). Survivors may dissociate and not hear the teacher when they ask about comfort levels with physical assists. Survivors may also dissociate throughout class when they are triggered.
- Assists can take away from survivors' being in the present moment and being in their own bodies.
- For some survivors, physical assists may be very healing, especially if they have a supportive relationship with the teacher. But it is critical to ask every single time—no matter how advanced the class is and no matter how many times the student has been in class with you.
- For yoga instructors teaching in the community, it is important to remember that there are survivors in your yoga classes every single day. Many survivors love their heated vinyasa flow, boot-camp classes, and so on, and also have clear emotional and physical boundaries and want to be in spaces where those are respected. For some survivors, it may be about cultivating a trusting relationship with the teacher before they are comfortable with physical assists.
- I invite you to think about the student's experience versus the teacher's expectation of how the class will unfold. Sometimes we go into class with a very specific sequence and idea of how

we want the class to look, how we want to set up a certain inversion, or how we want students to be in their bodies. But the most powerful experience is when a survivor can decide for themselves what feels right in their own body.

- Oftentimes the students who want to set boundaries the most are the least likely to communicate them. This is an important lens for each of us to hold in our respective professional roles so we can be intentional when creating a consent policy for assists.

- We have such a powerful opportunity to teach students about their capacity to self- and co-regulate, tap into their inner resilience, and help them recognize that within their body they have all of the tools for healing and that they don't have to do it alone. And the beauty of this is that we can provide this support without ever offering a hands-on assist.

- Some survivors are not ready to be seen and do not want the extra attention on them through a physical assist.

- Consider the way that trauma manifests in the body. Many of us have trauma stored in different parts of our bodies, depending on the nature of the assault. It is important to honor the modifications that students make in class and avoid prescriptive cues. This testimonial from Margaret Howard's article in the *Huffington Post* demonstrates this in a powerful way:

*Once, a yoga teacher insisted that I put my foot on my ankle in Vrksasana, tree pose. I didn't know why at that moment, but I really, really didn't want to. I could see the back of her shoulders tense up and hear her voice tighten as she continued to "suggest" I just "try it her way." But I was very happy and comfortable with my foot on my thigh, and very uncomfortable involving my ankle. A couple of years went by, then bam! the other day I made the connection, in a session with my own trauma therapist. That ankle is the one I broke when I was 11 years old. There is trauma held there. No wonder I didn't want to do that, the therapist said. Touching an area that holds trauma can, again, activate that trauma.* (Howard, 2013)

**Additional Recommendations:**

- Consider changing your assist policy to invite students who do want physical assists to "opt in." This removes the burden from the student to communicate no and applies the concept of consent to the yoga space.

- Integrate choice-based and empowering language throughout the entire class, to be mindful of student experiences with dissociation.

- Please ask about physical assists every single class. Students come to class with a different story every single day. There are many ways to ask! One of my favorite tools is the Yoga Flip-Chip because of the fluidity it creates in the practice. A survivor can say, "It is okay here, but not here" by flipping their chip, with Non-assist and Assist on either side. **This gives them agency and choice to change their mind at any time.**

- Body language is a powerful indicator of comfort. Pay attention to facial expression, rigid body posture and gestures, a startle response, shallow breathing, dissociation (or disengagement from the body), or lack of eye contact, to name a few. The nonverbal communication from your students may communicate more than words.

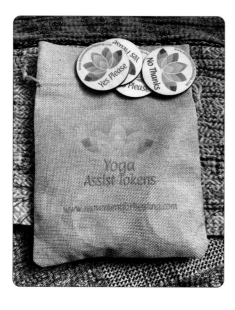

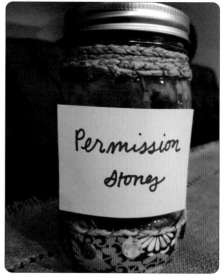

- Be creative with the various ways you are inviting students to exercise choice in class. See the images below for examples of permission stones, yoga assist tokens, and consent cards.

Lastly, while there are so many sensitivities to tend to and nurture, remember that survivors are incredibly resilient and strong—not fragile. The more choice you offer them, the more space and opportunity you create for them to fully embody their innate resilience, power, and control.

## 5. Creating Safety in the Physical Yoga Space

"Neuroception" is a term that comes from the work of Stephen Porges and describes how "neural circuits distinguish whether a situation is safe, threatening, or dangerous. It is the process in which our autonomic nervous system evaluates information from our senses about our environment and state of our body" (Rosenberg, 2017). It is essentially how we can determine whether the environment we are in is safe. I want to invite you to think about a survivor who might be new to the practice of yoga. Maybe someone recommends it to them as a way to help them manage their anxiety or depression. Maybe they have never practiced before and

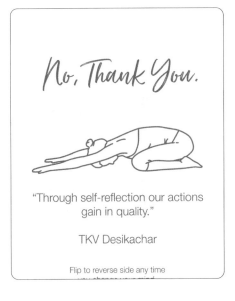

No, Thank You.

"Through self-reflection our actions gain in quality."

TKV Desikachar

Flip to reverse side any time

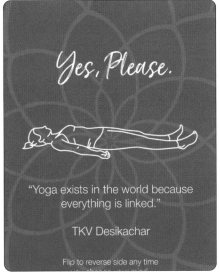

Yes, Please.

"Yoga exists in the world because everything is linked."

TKV Desikachar

Flip to reverse side any time

don't have a lot of context regarding what to look for. Perhaps they go to the first class they can find. Imagine what it might be like for them walking into a yoga space or studio for the first time. Perhaps they see straps hanging on the wall, they notice people are wearing minimal clothing, they see that there is not a lot of space between mats in the room, and that the room is very hot—making it difficult to regulate their temperature. Perhaps when the class begins, the teacher places hands on them without their permission. Can you see how suddenly a place they hoped would feel safe and supportive has become harmful and triggering?

As with everything discussed in this book thus far, it is important to invite survivors to have control over the environment of the physical class space as well. There are so many mindful shifts we can explore to help make the space more comfortable and accessible. Students who live with ongoing trauma symptoms and PTSD can be sensitive to sounds, temperature, and physical proximity, among many other elements. Changes in language and empowering agency throughout class can support survivors in working toward an internal and external sense of safety in the room.

But first, I just want to take a moment to **pause and check in with you**.

I remember in one of my in-person trainings, I noticed that one of the participants had a distressed expression on her face. During the break I checked in with her to see how she was doing. She shared that she was afraid that she was going to cause more harm in her classes. As we connected, it reminded me of a quote I had read from Lisa Danylchuk (2019): "We cannot prevent all experiences that activate a negative samskara, or traumatic memory. Instead we seek to create an embodied experience of safety, and when triggers arise, offer support through the tools we have learned." I shared this with her and reminded her about the power of her healing presence. That this alone would have a tremendous impact on the way she held space for survivors. My sincere hope is that you don't get too caught up in the checklist. This is your invitation to be attuned to the survivors who are in front of you, because they really are your greatest teachers. These tools are meant to be a supportive place for you to land, to have in your toolbox, and to refer back to when you need extra support.

Consider the lives you impact and the healing that happens when you affirm, acknowledge, and speak to those holding the most vulnerable experiences in the room. When we prioritize those voices, we create spaces where survivors feel seen. We communicate that their experiences matter and that they are not invisible. Some of you may be facilitating closed classes for survivors of sexual assault, others might be integrating some of the tools into community classes, and perhaps others are finding ways to integrate these tools into clinical practice, teaching spaces, or outreach work. Below are some ways you might increase safety in the physicality of the spaces in which you are teaching or offering these tools:

- Invite students to set up wherever they would like and empower them to make changes as they see fit. Provide multiple options to increase comfort (e.g., sitting in a chair, using bolsters and blankets, etc.).
- Be mindful of the use of straps in trauma-informed classes. They can be triggering for a survivor who has past trauma that involves being bound or immobilized in some capacity. If I am teaching in a space that has them, I typically store them away.
- Connect with students about the temperature in the room. Ask them how it feels and what adjustments can be made to increase comfort. Be mindful of the lighting in the room and avoid candles or replace them with translucent options.
- Consider playing instrumental or neutral music.
- Help orient students to the space so they know where the exit doors are and how to safely access those options.
- When I notice there are unexpected noises arising in the space, whether due to late arrivals or loud sounds from outside, I do my best to name what is happening. The same goes if I have to move around the room to adjust the lighting or music or for any other reason. It helps to remove any element of surprise and informs students of where you are in the space.

- As best as you can, try to be flexible with late arrivals. Perhaps integrate this into your language to help prepare everyone for what that might look like. **So often showing up is the hardest part.**

## 6. A Trauma-Sensitive Approach to Breath Work and Mindfulness

*Your breath is the voice of your body. . . . Your breath has a story to tell.*
—DR. GAIL PARKER, *RESTORATIVE YOGA FOR ETHNIC AND RACE-BASED STRESS AND TRAUMA*

In her book *Trauma and the Body*, Pat Ogden (2006) shares how those who have experienced trauma "often experience inner-body sensations as overwhelming or distressing." As a result, breath work and mindfulness-meditation practices can trigger traumatic experiences and memories for survivors in many different ways. In her book *Attachment-Based Yoga and Meditation for Trauma Recovery*, Deirdre Fay (2017) shares, "There are times when trauma clients feel swallowed by the intensity of their symptoms, unable to separate from them." And telling students to "just breathe and sit with it" or pay close attention to their breath and inner sensations when they are struggling during yoga or mindfulness practice can actually exacerbate their symptoms of traumatic stress. Caitlin Lanier (2019), trauma-informed yoga instructor and LCSW, says it is dangerous for us to assume that "all yoga practices, including breath work, are inherently healing and helpful for trauma survivors." For example, imagine what it might feel like if your breath feels choppy or panicky and then you are asked to engage in a specific breathing practice, at a very particular pace or number count. There have been many times during my yoga practice when the breath cues have overwhelmed my nervous system, similar to the way my trauma symptoms do. *I want to invite you to take a pause here and engage with your breath at a pace that feels comfortable to you. There is absolutely no rush. Take all the time you need. If it feels supportive, you might place one palm over your heart, and one palm over your belly, and notice the rise and fall of your beautiful breath. With compassionate awareness, honor all that you do, all that you are, all that you hold. You are enough, just as you are.*

Breath can be linked to past experiences of trauma, especially as we consider the different elements of traumatic experiences: holding the breath, accelerated heart rate, constricted breathing, inability to breathe, shortness of breath, suffocation (Turner & Emerson, personal communication, October 28, 2012). When breath work is taught in a way that is activating or triggering, it has the potential to flood survivors with emotional memories. In his book *Overcoming Trauma Through Yoga*, Emerson (2011) writes, "When the survival response is activated, breathing often becomes more rapid and shallow, increasing oxygen throughout the body. . . . When they are triggered or overwhelmed, many trauma survivors also tend to hold their breath, often unconsciously." The holding of the breath in many cases can be protection from emotions that are too painful to be with and is "a learned response to stress, anxiety, feeling scared, and the presence of difficult sensations and emotions" (Patterson, 2020). Nityda Gessel, founder of the Trauma-Conscious Yoga Institute, shares some additional ways survivors may be triggered by focusing on their breath:

- "If our trauma involved being unable to breathe or fighting for our breath.
- If we felt our life was in danger (remember the breath involves not only the bringing in, but also the exiting of the life force or prana).
- If we are frozen in a hyper-aroused, or fight-or-flight state (unfortunately, people who have experienced prolonged exposure to stress and trauma can become stuck here and some people who are chronically here will not find relief in deep breathing)."

(Gessel, 2018)

Just like the healing process, the regulation of one's nervous system takes time and support. Ultimately, the hope is that the breath can feel more spacious and restorative instead of triggering. And this is absolutely possible with time and patience, as well as with gentle, compassionate, trauma-informed instruction.

## BENEFITS OF TRAUMA-INFORMED BREATH WORK AND MEDITATION

One of the most supportive things we can do when offering breath work or meditation practice is provide survivors with adequate space and choices to engage with their breath in a way that feels safe, accessible, and on their terms. Many folks ask me if this means they should not offer a specific breath practice, such as ujjayi breath, breath of fire, lion's breath, or alternate nostril (to name a few). And that always brings me back to the box we discussed at the beginning of the book. There is no one-size-fits-all approach. Please continue to offer breath practices, but consider providing choices within those options to modify or opt out, to support a survivor's sense of safety and ability to self- or co-regulate in a way that feels manageable. There are a number of therapeutic benefits to engaging with the breath, including a tangible practice to support nervous system regulation; the opportunity it provides to practice self-compassion, self-care, and presence; and the way it helps invite both calming and energizing feelings into the body. Additional improvements linked with physical and mental health include decreases in PTSD, anxiety, stress, GI issues, chronic pain, and depression; and increases in sleep, coping skills, resilience, energy, and overall health.

Below are some ways to be mindful of how you might offer these practices in a trauma-informed way. You may also find the section on supporting students who are triggered later in this chapter to be helpful in supplementing this information. It helps to provide more context for how to support students when they may be experiencing activating, triggering, or intense physiological symptoms.

## WATCH FOR DYSREGULATED AROUSAL

It is helpful to first have a lens of what to look for if a student is triggered in class or if the meditation or breath work may be harming rather than helping. In his book *Trauma-Sensitive Mindfulness*, David Treleaven outlines the following ways to watch for dysregulated arousal during mindfulness practice:

- *Muscle tone extremely slack (collapsed, noticeably flat affect)*
- *Muscle tone extremely rigid*
- *Hyperventilation*
- *Exaggerated startle response*
- *Excessive sweating*
- *Noticeable dissociation (person appears highly disconnected from their body)*
- *Noticeably pale skin tone*
- *Emotional volatility (enraged, excessive crying, terror)*
- *Disorganized speech or slurring words*
- *Reports of blurred vision*
- *Inability to make eye contact*
- *Reports of flashbacks, nightmares or intrusive thoughts*

(Treleaven, 2018)

Additionally, in my work with sexual assault survivors, the ways I have seen triggers manifest in the practice space have included hypervigilance, fear, irritability and agitation, moving around the room, paranoia, nausea, fatigue, and panic attacks.

## OFFER A VARIETY OF CUES AND CHOICES TO ENGAGE WITH THE BREATH

*Examples might include:*

"I invite you to breathe in and out at your pace. You are welcome to explore one of the breath practices I am about to share and you can go at your pace. There is absolutely no rush. If you find that the practice does not feel supportive for you, you can opt out at any time or explore these additional modifications: [x, y, z]."

"Throughout our practice you are welcome to keep your eyes open, find a soft gaze, or close them if that feels comfortable for you. Know that your choices are celebrated here."

"If it feels right for you, you could explore resting one hand on your belly and one hand on your heart. How does it feel to notice the rise and fall of your breath? Take your time. I invite you to come into your breath on your terms. You can make a change or opt out at any time. This is your practice and always your choice."

**Additional tools to explore integrating into your classes when offering trauma-informed breath options:**

- Create a culture of consent.
- Encourage and empower survivors to integrate movement into a meditation practice if stillness is too triggering (i.e., if rest does not feel safe).
- Make modifications in the physical space to create safety.
- Have a plan to support students who are triggered during the practice. See section on supporting students who are triggered later in this chapter for further guidance and support.
- Have a safety and consent protocol for entering a student's personal space.
- Utilize baseline cards or arousal scales as an ongoing form of assessment. This provides a tangible way to invite survivors to practice embodied check-ins and provide feedback about the impact the practice may be having on their healing process. This will be further discussed in Chapter 5 in the section on understanding assessment and liability.

## LEADING A TRAUMA-INFORMED BODY SCAN
## AND SAVASANA

I invite you to revisit the section on empowerment-based language in this chapter and also apply this to leading body scans and savasana. When working with survivors of sexual assault, please be mindful of areas of the body that may be particularly sensitive or hold trauma memories (pelvic area, thighs, buttocks). Additionally, as shared earlier in this chapter in the section on consent and physical assists in yoga spaces survivors hold trauma in various parts of their bodies depending on the nature of what they have experienced. And the most empowering thing we can do is provide choices and opportunities to opt out of what does not feel comfortable. Again, please be mindful about asking survivors to engage in certain contemplative practices that do not feel supportive for them or their healing, as these can worsen their symptoms of traumatic stress.

While we often think of savasana as one of the most relaxing parts of the practice, there are a number of reasons it can be an incredibly challenging posture for survivors. This may include the darkness of the room; the inability to know where the teacher is in the space and whether they may come over to offer an assist; being told to close the eyes or not to move as the only option; and the challenges of being still when experiencing trauma symptoms, PTSD, and/or dissociation.

It can take all the strength in the world for survivors to have the courage to get to their mat. As discussed in Chapter 1, it is important to be aware of the ongoing impact of tonic immobility or rape-induced paralysis. Savasana can bring on an onset of triggers associated with the freeze response.

Your language is powerful. Take time to provide a number of different options and empower students to find what feels best. Remind them they can change their mind at any time.

- Rest is deeply personal and you are always in choice around what feels best for you. I invite you to find a final savasana that supports your body. Know that you could explore one shape and shift at any time to increase your comfort. You could explore any of the following options or any other shape that resonates with you:

- Perhaps explore lying on your side and using any props to support your body. They are there as a resource—keeping you lifted and held.

- If you'd like, you could explore lying on your belly and resting your head on your hands.

- You always have the option to close your practice in a seated meditation with your eyes open, closed, or finding a soft gaze. Find any variation that feels comfortable to you.

- It might feel nice to lie on your back and bring the soles of your feet to the mat. If you'd like you could rest your knees together.

- If it feels safe for you, you could explore resting on your back and placing one hand on your belly and one hand on your heart.

- You are *always in choice, and you can start with any of these options and make a change at any time. This is your body, your practice, and always your choice.*

**Additional factors to consider when leading a trauma-informed savasana:**

- Explore safe and supportive lighting options.
- Remind students they can leave the room at any time.
- Have a consent framework for assists, touch, use of essential oils, and so on.
- Welcome movement instead of just stillness.
- Provide multiple options for each student (as shared above) to explore their own unique savasana. This might include seated meditation, lying on side or belly, sitting in a chair, legs up the wall, resting hands on belly and heart, and so on.
- Invite students to keep their eyes open or find a soft gaze.
- Lastly, please do not take photos of your students during savasana (or at any point in class). This is a sacred time and practice and students are trusting you with their safety and confidentiality.

If you would like additional guidance, Molly Boeder Harris (Boeder Harris, 2015) has a wonderful video on YouTube titled *Trauma-Informed Savasana*.

## MINDFULNESS MEDITATION AS AN ONGOING RESOURCE: A PERSONAL PRACTICE

As a survivor, I have learned indirectly through my mindfulness-meditation practice to passionately take in moments of joy. To hold them and honor them, in the moment, just as they are. To cherish them and savor them, no matter how fleeting. And to let that part of the practice spill over into all aspects of my life—serving as a continual resource and, in many cases, capacity and resilience builder.

# A framework for ensuring your classes are more trauma-informed

What if, together, we could reenvision healing spaces in this world? If every yoga instructor and studio:

..................

Knew that there were survivors taking their classes every single day. That many of their students are coping with PTSD, anxiety, and depression. And that often their symptoms have continued to permeate their lived experience long after the trauma(s) occurred.

..................

Affirmed their students just for showing up. Because we all know that so often that is the hardest part.

..................

Knew that being trauma informed should not be optional.

..................

Knew that the diversity of their teaching staff matters.

..................

Used invitational and empowering language so students were reminded often that they are enough exactly as they are.

..................

Reminded students of the power of celebrating the choices they have with their own bodies.

..................

Asked themselves who they are not seeing come through their doors and why that is. And what changes could they begin making to create a more inclusive, safer environment?

Applied the concepts of consent to the studio environment and every class they teach. What if each class was a celebration of the physical and emotional boundaries of their students?

..................

Could learn about trauma in their 200-hour teacher training.

..................

Integrated trauma-sensitive breath options to support survivors in the inherent triggers related to breath work.

..................

Provided a variety of options for resting in savasana and were mindful of the common triggers related to the freeze response.

..................

Reminded students that they can leave class at any time.

..................

Had a plan for supporting students with triggers.

..................

Used gender-neutral language and asked about pronouns.

..................

Were intentional about creating spaces for all bodies, folks in the LGBTQ community, other marginalized groups, and people of every race, socioeconomic status, and gender identity.

..................

Had gender-neutral bathrooms and safe spaces for people to change in.

..................

Had a consent-affirming assist policy.

..................

Were reminded frequently that their healing matters, too.

# Trauma-Informed Yoga Language Reframes

| INSTEAD OF | PERHAPS TRY THIS |
| --- | --- |
| Using gendered language in your yoga classes | Ask about pronouns and use inclusive language ("folks," "all," "friends"). |
| Appropriating cultural practices in yoga | Do your research about the origins of ancient healing traditions. |
| Adjusting or correcting someone when they choose their own variation of the posture | Consider the way students hold trauma in various parts of their bodies. Trust your students as they make choices that best serve them. |
| Picking a quote to read without much thought | Be intentional. Reading poems and quotes from people of color means more than you know. |
| Telling students to close their eyes as the only option, to sit still, or to stay in the room the entire time | Remember that this can evoke trauma symptoms and triggers of the freeze response. Please be mindful of the ways you can create safety in your classes for all. |
| Using very prescriptive cues | You can't remind survivors enough about the choices they have with their own bodies. |
| Offering physical assists without permission | Please don't. Always have a consent protocol for assists. |
| Offering a single disclaimer at the beginning of class about resting, invitations, or opting out | Integrate that language throughout the entire class, especially given how common dissociation is. |
| Thinking there is a specific checklist to being more trauma informed | This work requires a lifelong commitment of learning and putting survivors at the center of their own experience. |
| Telling students to stay in the room the entire time and drink water only at the designated breaks | "You are welcome to leave the room at any time and drink water as you need. Your comfort and safety are the most important elements of your practice." |

# Trauma-Informed Yoga Language Reframes

| INSTEAD OF | PERHAPS TRY THIS |
| --- | --- |
| Using very specific breath practices | Remember that breath work can trigger traumatic experiences and memories in many different ways. Provide students with options to breathe in ways that feel comfortable for them. |
| "Lie on your back and be still" | "You are worthy and welcome to explore what savasana looks like in your body." (Offer many posture options and affirm that movement is okay.) |
| Using "push harder" language | Yoga is a practice that began in India as a means to transcend suffering. Life is hard enough—our practice doesn't have to be. |
| Thinking trauma-informed frameworks don't apply to your teaching style | Be mindful that there are multiple students in class who have experienced trauma and as a result may suffer from the physical and emotional symptoms that still permeate their lived experience long after the incident(s) occurred. Healing is not linear. |
| "Just sit with it" | If students are flooded with emotional or painful memories during meditation, remind them it is okay to stop or opt out. Have a plan to support students who are triggered. |
| "I don't offer a lot of breaks in class." | "I invite you to honor the wisdom of your body and take breaks whenever you need. I celebrate the intentional choices you make for you. Resting is a beautiful choice. You are your greatest teacher and you are enough just as you are." |

When I stopped treating meditation as another thing I needed to fit into my schedule, it created small, but empowering shifts in my life, the day-to-day, and my healing process. I am certainly human and meditation is an ongoing practice, but whether it's intentionally taking a deep breath and dropping into my body before giving a big speech, taking in a hug from my son in the most mindful of ways, choosing to close my computer and my eyes, resting a palm on my heart and belly instead of powering through, savoring a cup of coffee—there are so many ways that weaving the practice into my day has changed my life. The resources are within us and around us.

Some of my most mindful moments are when I am immersed in nature with my family. During the COVID-19 pandemic especially, I will remember the daily hikes in Los Angeles with my husband and our time spent among the trees chasing our 3-year-old son and hearing his sweet belly laughs. There are days I stare at him and see the way he laughs with his whole entire body and all I feel in that moment is pure joy and presence. I will remember our drives down the Pacific Coast Highway watching the waves and seeing my son's face light up as he gazed out the window. I hold sweet memories of him sprinting in the sand as we watched a gorgeous sunset and then gently putting his toes in the ocean. I will remember our long walks picking up fall leaves and wondering if he would always hold my hand that way. I will remember our collective exhale breath. Nature has that ability to ground us, remind us of the preciousness of each moment, embody joy, and return us to ourselves.

Because the thing is, the waves of life are strong and smooth and then they repeat. And none of us are immune from the next wave or the next storm. And you deserve anchoring, joyful, restful moments wherever you can grasp them. These are the moments when our practice inevitably intersects with what may feel like ordinary moments. But with intention, they have the capacity to provide resourcing in profound ways.

## 7. Supporting Students Who Are Triggered

I want to invite you to take a moment and rest a palm on your heart and a palm on your belly. I invite you to notice the rise and fall of your breath. Follow its lead here for as long as it feels comfortable to you. Please know that it is impossible to tend to every emotion and potential trigger that might arise when offering trauma-informed yoga, but there are tools to help equip you to feel more confident, grounded, and supported. Triggers are a normal part of the healing journey and it can be powerful when a survivor learns tools to help them regain control on their own terms and at their own pace. For example, I was working with a survivor who often had to see her perpetrator on campus. Prior to participating in the trauma-informed yoga program, she would understandably feel incredibly triggered when she saw them, and it would often send her into a depressive state. She told me that each time an encounter would happen, she would return to her dorm room and not leave for a few days. This made her academic environment incredibly unsafe. She didn't feel quite comfortable accessing other resources on campus, but over the course of the program, she learned tools that allowed her to feel safely embodied. She gained her strength, courage, and power back. She reminded herself often that she was worthy of choices and that she had a right to feel safe on her campus. Whenever she would see her perpetrator, she would take a moment to sit down and place her hands over her heart and belly. She would journal about how she was feeling to affirm how valid her feelings of anger were. She would repeat positive affirmations to herself to increase her sense of safety and would practice specific mudras to help her feel protected. She would take a moment to notice her feet on the ground and practice exercises to bring her into the present moment. She would explore turning the volume of her heart up and the volume of her thoughts down. She slowly learned how to reclaim her body and her space. The practices could never take away the pain and suffering that individual caused her, but they did support her in loosening the grip that the trauma had on her heart.

Below are some tools to support you with helping manage triggers that might arise when facilitating a trauma-informed yoga class:

- Before you begin the practice, you might have a discussion with students about what it would look like to identify an inner resource, a supportive mantra, an anchor, or an intention they feel connected to. Perhaps this can be what they focus on when painful memories or triggers begin to arise in the body.

- Remember that body language is a strong indicator of someone's comfort level in class. Dr. Lisa Lewis (2021) quotes Laura Khoudari and shares, "Pay attention to what your client's body is saying and not just what they are saying with their words. This is a technique called 'tracking.'" This can give you information about their comfort levels and when it may be appropriate to check in.

- I invite you to take some time to develop a tool kit of exercises that you can draw from to assist students with managing triggers, as it may not be the best time to introduce something new. Examples might include Mountain Pose, grounding seated postures, and/or repeated sun salutations (with various options for all).

- Explore offering self-regulating and self-soothing postures. Examples include hands on belly and heart to notice and feel each inhale and exhale, Adi Mudra, Bhu Mudra, Butterfly Hug, and Peter Levine's 5-Step Self-Holding Exercise to name a few.

- If being with the internal sensations feels too overwhelming, you might invite students to reorient by focusing on what is happening outside the body—touch, taste, smell, sight, hearing: also known as exteroceptive sensations.

- You can invite students to bring a grounding object to class to support them when triggered. Examples include a stone, crystal, fidget cube, pipe cleaner, and so on.

- You can always invite students to open their eyes at any time or take a break from the activity, exercise, or posture.

- If you are offering the program at a specific agency/university, it can be helpful to have a release/exchange of information with a survivor's therapist advocate, to be able to work collaboratively to support the student.
- Know that triggers will inevitably arise, despite your best intentions. Be prepared to stay grounded, calm, and present with the entire class.
- Allow for tears and expression of feelings and understand that trauma may affect a survivor's response. There is no "normal" way to process the impact of trauma. Respect their individual journey.
- Empower the survivor to make their own decisions, and ASK what you can do to be supportive.
- Be prepared with additional support resources for survivors who can support them in ways that are beyond your scope of practice. Examples include hotline numbers, support groups, rape crisis centers, survivor advocates, local trauma therapists, and holistic healing options.
- Invite students to listen to the wisdom of their own bodies and be gentle with their experience. Remind them that their emotions are valid and welcome.
- Invite the inquiries: What is coming up for me and what do I need? What does this moment require?
- Invite students to connect with something tangible. Example: "Take a moment to notice the support of the mat or the seat beneath you. What would it feel like to allow yourself to feel held? Know that you are supported and that you are never alone in your experience."
- Invite students to couple an affirmation that resonates with them with a yoga posture (e.g., "I am grounded in my truth" with Tree Pose/Vrksasana). See Chapter 6 for more examples of yoga postures coupled with affirmations.

## 8. Cultural Considerations and Accessibility

*Yoga, historically a system for healing and liberation, trains us to inhabit our bodies through mindful movements. Many of these healing practices originated in indigenous traditions, yet such support is rarely accessible to marginalized people who most need it. It is time to change that. It is time to demand the freedoms and opportunity to heal our bodies as a human right. It is time to organize not just around our trauma but around our collective healing.*
—VALARIE KAUR, *SEE NO STRANGER*


*Yes, individual healing practices might be helpful in managing trauma, but they are incomplete and inadequate without addressing the broader systemic injustices that can traumatize so many.*
—HALA KHOURI, *PEACE FROM ANXIETY*


### A PERSONAL CONNECTION TO EMBODIED INEQUALITY

One of my first visceral experiences with racism was in high school shortly after the tragedy of 9/11, when one of my classmates stopped me in the hallway when I was walking to class, put his hand on my shoulder, and told me that it was probably my dad who was flying the plane. I remember feeling completely frozen and disembodied. I wanted to shrink, hide, and crawl out of my skin. I was triggered before I even really understood what that word actually meant, or what it would come to mean years later in the aftermath of surviving sexual assault and the loss of a child.

These experiences and encounters continued over the years in the form of microaggressions, sexism, dehumanization, and other forms of belittling. One of the most recent experiences was last year, when I was hired to be a trainer and the landlord of the building where I was facilitating the training told me I was unwelcome in his break room and told me to remove my food from his refrigerator. I remember the hate and disgust in his eyes. I didn't eat that day for nearly 8 hours while facilitating a training on trauma (and ironically discussing how the impact of embodied inequality and race-based trauma can be similar to PTSD). When I finally got to the airport to head back to Los Angeles, I collapsed to the ground and sobbed hysterically. A security guard helped me up and expressed his genuine concern. All weekend I had suppressed all that pain and built-up oppression (and likely many years of memories and suppressed experiences), and suddenly my body could release it safely through the tears.

These experiences I have had over the years have without a doubt shaped who I trust, where I feel safe, my complex and nuanced relationship with my body, and my resilience. They felt important to include here in framing the ways our lived experiences shape how we show up to our practice and all the things we carry. When I think about these moments that so many of us navigate, it reminds me of a quote I have seen in many different forms over the years: "Just because we carry it well doesn't mean it's not heavy."

## CREATING AN INCLUSIVE ENVIRONMENT

In her book *Restorative Yoga for Ethnic and Race-Based Stress and Trauma*, Dr. Gail Parker (2020) shares that "many people feel uncomfortable entering yoga studios, because it is just one more place where they risk being invalidated, rendered invisible, or treated as other." It is critical that, as folks sharing this practice with survivors, we root ourselves in the framework of Ahimsa. Being an ally is committing to showing up and helping people feel seen, welcomed, cared for, and enough. There are many moments when, as I write and prepare for classes or workshops, I sit quietly and hold space in my heart and thoughts for those who hold the most vulnerable experiences. I think about all the survivors of color who have participated in the trauma-informed yoga series and shared that it was one of the first places they felt seen and safe and felt like they could breathe with ease and take up space. The power of trauma-informed and culturally affirming collective movement is that oftentimes there are just no words—the connection is felt. Communities who have been historically marginalized deserve supportive tools for nervous system regulation as they navigate daily experiences of systemic oppression and ongoing trauma resulting in embodied inequality. They are worthy of rest. They deserve affirming community and reminders of their resilience.

We are so lucky to have incredibly informative resources and tools readily available to us to support our learning as trauma-informed practitioners. This self-work, learning, and unlearning are critical to every aspect of our lifelong commitment as practitioners and allies. We must also remind ourselves often that our bodies weren't designed to integrate this material quickly. In the age of information, it is likely that our nervous systems are on high alert all the time. We must move slowly in order for change to be sustainable, and prioritize moments of compassion and rest whenever possible. Allow the necessary time for integration. I have included additional resources to support your learning in the appendix, including a list of incredible educators doing social-justice activism work in yoga.

The concepts of cultural considerations, intersectionality, social justice, and accessibility could be a training and book all on their own. But anytime we are discussing the trauma of sexual assault, we must also remember how imperative it is to be rooted in racial justice. Audre Lorde's (1982) words have carried my heart amid this work: "There is no such thing as a single-issue struggle because we do not live single-issue lives." When we approach the work from an "intersectional lens," a term coined by Dr. Kimberlé Crenshaw, we also provide different pathways for survivors who hold various marginalized and intersecting identities to access healing. There are already many barriers to the practice for survivors who are people of color, LGBTQ, undocumented, refugees and immigrants, veterans, or homeless, and for those representing a diversity of body shapes and abilities. When we center their experiences in the scope of our work, we can create programs, services, and healing spaces that are more inclusive and intentional.

There is not a one-size-fits-all approach. Survivors need and deserve to come to classes and feel that they belong and that their experiences matter. Jocelyn Frye and colleagues (2019) share how systemic biases perpetuate gender-based based violence and this is often left out of the conversation. This includes biases based on race, sex, ethnicity, gender identity, sexual orientation, religion, national origin, and disability. All of these identities shape a survivor's holistic experience, lens, and access (or lack thereof) to traditional support services. Additionally, survivors who hold intersecting and marginalized identities not only experience higher rates of sexual assault but are often left out of the broader national discussions of these issues, which leads to further invisibility and minimization of their experiences.

Survivors who identify as women of color are only "half to one third as likely as their white counterparts to seek mental health services following trauma" (Harris & Linder, 2017). In their study on the specific experiences of 34 women of color who are survivors of sexual violence across multiple university settings, Harris, Karunaratne, and Gutzwa (in press) found that trauma-informed yoga had a significant impact on their healing. What follows is an excerpt from their study:

> For a majority of women in this study, "body-based work" was integral to their healing process. Body-based practices, also known as somatic therapy, is centered on bodily awareness and the body's connection to the mind (Levine, 2010). . . . Women often explored different types of body-based modalities for healing, such as ballet, running, and jiu-jitsu. Yet, the majority of women who named body-based work as a modality for healing participated in, and spoke about, the body-based practice of yoga. Women almost always connected their experiences with yoga as healing to a yoga program that existed at each institution. Each institution's yoga program was offered through the Sexual Violence Advocacy and Education Office and the programs were meant for participants to explore and re-gain control of their bodies after trauma.

*Samantha, a Mexican/Vietnamese woman, recalled, "I did [the institution's] eight-week yoga session and now all I do is meditate. I love meditating. It's perfect. It really just helps me. It's helped me heal so much." Leya, a half Black/half Pakistani woman, explained in more detail why she found yoga, and the yoga program, to be a "helpful" healing space: I did the [yoga program at this institution] and that was when I actually really fell in love with it. And that's when it really started to help. It was because it was such a safe space, and I had not been in a safe space in so long. It was addicting to be in that safe space. As a follow-up to her statement, the lead researcher asked, "What makes it a safe space?" Leya replied: It's probably the instructor telling us that we can do whatever we want to do when we come into the room. We can take a nap, we can talk, we could not talk. We participate, we cannot participate. We can do all the poses or if a pose is uncomfortable you can stop. It's like someone telling us we have the freedom to not go along. . . . All the other girls also being uncomfortable was also very comfortable, because we all knew that we all have been through something. And it was a unity in silence thing because no one wants to talk about it because we weren't there to talk about it. We were there to go into ourselves. It wasn't supposed to be a therapy session. I really liked that. (Harris et al., in press)*

Below are a few considerations to begin integrating into your own education as an ally, into your classes and spaces, and into your teaching instruction, to help all survivors feel seen.

- **Make a plan for survivors with diverse abilities.** One day when I was teaching, a student came to class in a wheelchair. In my most honest moment, I felt incredibly nervous. I wanted to do everything in my power to ensure the class was supportive and inclusive. I took a deep breath and gazed over my sequence for class. I made notes to myself and adjusted the sequence structure to ensure that the student felt seen and could safely move through the practice in community with her peers. After the practice she shared with me that it was one of the first times in a yoga space that she did not feel invisible. As many times as I second-guessed myself, I couldn't help but feel emotional when thinking about the power of centering her experience. Spend some time thinking about the accessibility of your classes. Don't be afraid to ask your students what they need. Have chairs available and supportive props for people who cannot sit on yoga mats.

- **Create accessible and inclusive spaces.** I invite you to think back to the framework of supportive presence. What other factors might contribute to students feeling comfortable in the actual yoga space? Are there gender-neutral bathrooms and safe places for people to change in? Is there signage or imagery that reflects an inclusive community?

- **Provide accommodations.** Spend some time in communication with studio owners of the space where you teach to discuss accommodations for students and explore integrating inclusive language on the website. Consider various factors such as learning disorders, traumatic brain injury, psychological disorders, physical and mobility impairments, and sensory impairments. Accessible Yoga is a wonderful organization that provides many resources and training to further your study in this area.

- **Create financial accessibility.** In whatever capacity works for you, offer sliding-scale spots, scholarships, and/or donation-based classes to increase access.

- **Explain Sanskrit.** Trauma-informed approaches are intentional about honoring the roots of the practice.

- **Use gender-neutral language.** Examples include addressing students as "folks," "all," and "friends." Ask your students about their pronouns.

- **All bodies are different.** Avoid calling postures "easy." We know that there is no one-size-fits-all approach to the practice. Provide multiple options to create an inclusive space for those with differently abled bodies and all body sizes and shapes.
- **Practice cultural humility.** This means being aware of your own privilege. Also be gentle with yourself, as you are not always going to get it right. Dr. Wendy Ashley talks about a concept known as reflexive attentiveness, which is allowing ourselves to lean into the discomfort of these conversations in order to commit to the lifelong work of being an ally (personal communication, June 12, 2018). We must ask ourselves often: Who are we not seeing in the room, and why is that? And what steps can we take to make our spaces more inclusive?
- **Consider the concept of intersectionality.** As shared previously, "intersectionality" is a term coined by Dr. Kimberlé Crenshaw. It is a concept often used in critical race theories to describe the ways in which various systems of oppression (including racism, sexism, homophobia, transphobia, ableism, xenophobia, and classism) are interconnected and cannot be examined separately from one another. Research shows that those who experience multiple forms of discrimination are also at risk for additional mental health concerns. Let this inform your work and how you hold space for survivors.
- **Stay informed.** A big part of allyship and our commitment to holding affirming and inclusive spaces is keeping on top of the news and overall political climate. In her Creating Culturally-Sensitive Healing Spaces teleseminar for The Breathe Network on August 2, 2015, Grace Poon Ghaffari talked about the importance of being aware of when there are hate or bias incidents against people that share your student's identity. This may impact their overall well-being, what they are carrying,

and how they show up to their practice. Take the time to check in with them to express your care and concern.

- **Include quotes, affirmations, or songs from people of color in your classes.** It means more than you know to hear those words and feel those identities reflected.

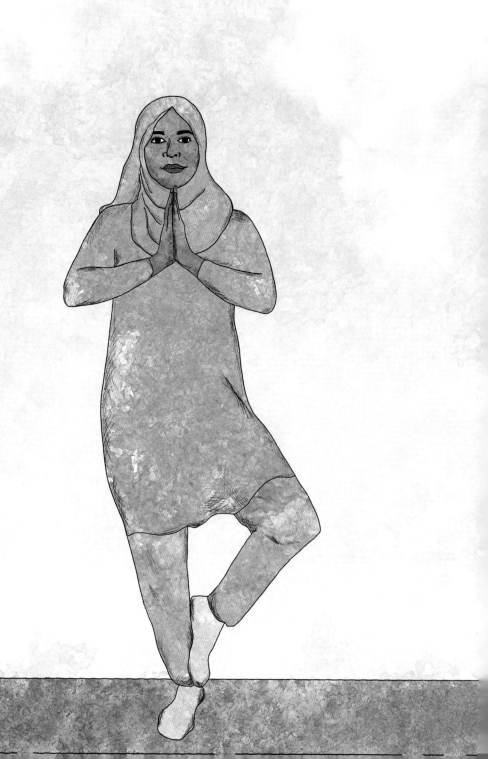

## ◆ 4 ◆

# Dear Survivors,
# Your Body Remembers.
# Be Gentle With You.

*i think it's brave that you get up in the morning even if your soul
is weary and your bones ache for a rest*

*i think it's brave that you keep on living
even if you don't know how to anymore*

*i think it's brave that you push away the waves rolling in every day
and you decide to fight
i know there are days when you feel like giving up but
i think it's brave
that you never do*
—LANA RAFAELA

*If you feel you've stalled or regressed in your healing, remember
the nervous system heals in waves of expansion and contraction.
2 to 3 steps forward, 1 step back. Just like muscles need rest
days your nervous system needs time for integration. Slow and
steady progress is sustainable.*
 —CASSANDRA SOLANO

Dear Survivor,

I am so grateful you are here. You are light. You are extraordinary. You are enough, exactly as you are. I invite you to take a moment and rest a palm over your heart and a palm over your belly. Perhaps feel the rise and fall of your breath. I invite you to breathe into your strength. The strength that has resided in your body all along. Maybe explore turning the volume of your heart up, and the volume of your thoughts all the way down. Perhaps explore noticing any areas of your body that are holding tension. Does it feel okay to send your breath there? Continue your breath in ways that feel safe and accessible to you. Take your time as you settle into the safety of your body. Perhaps notice what is supporting you. Can you take note of the embodied experience of being held? Take a moment to send yourself gratitude for all the ways you have survived and continue to survive. Your resilience inspires us all.

It takes courage to tend to your healing. Your body deserves to feel what it's like to not live in a constant state of survival and stress. You are worthy of rest. You deserve to feel the expansion of your breath. To honor what your body is communicating to you about what it needs moment to moment. To respond in ways that feel kind and compassionate to you. To find your anchors of safety. To remind yourself that you are your greatest teacher.

If you have made it this far in the book, I can imagine it has stirred a combination of many different emotions. Know that whatever you feel is okay, valid, and welcome here. You are worthy of honoring your feelings. Be gentle with all the ways your body remembers.

What might it look like in the ongoing practice to hold the many paradoxes of our healing? To honor the grief, but also make space for abundant joy. What does it feel like to ride the waves of healing as they come? What if we could lean into compassion when we tap into the deep knowing that there may be no finish line to this thing called healing. Can we hold on fiercely to our worthiness amid the many storms we will inevitably navigate in this life? Can we allow ourselves to be present with moments of relief and joy? And can we consciously practice self-love amid the growing, the healing, the learning?

You are not defined by your trauma. You are celebrated for all that you are, all that you give, and all that you do. Thank you for all the ways you show up for yourself every single day. It is an honor to be witness to your healing.

The world needs your voice. The world needs your gifts. The world needs your healing. The world needs you. Keep going.

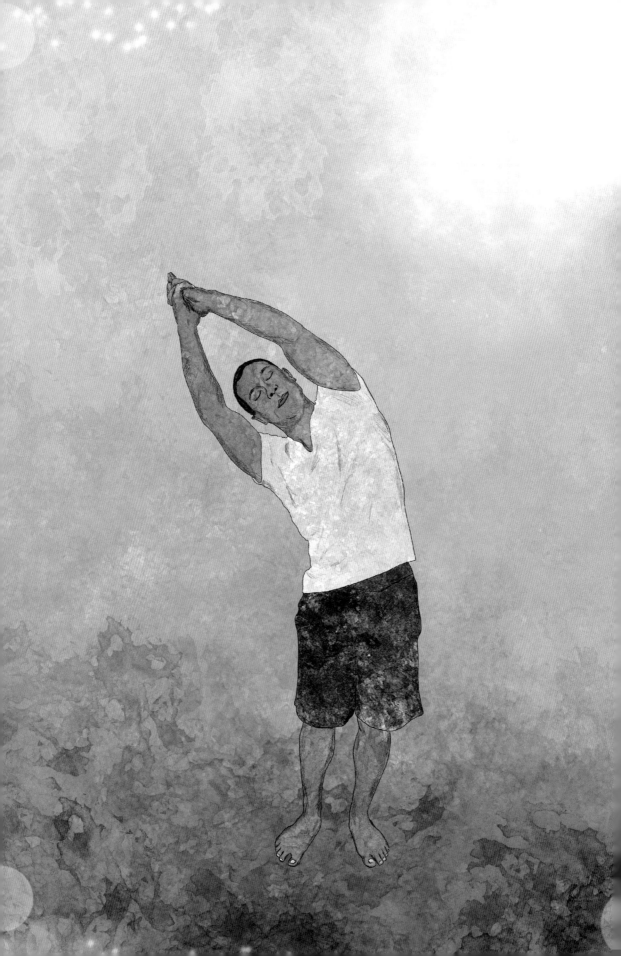

PART TWO

# Implementing a Trauma-Informed Framework

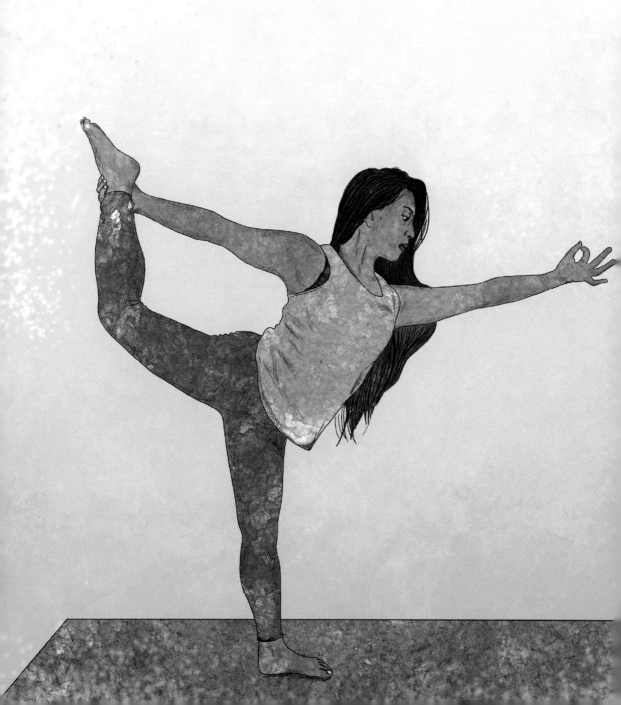

# ✦ 5 ✦

# Comprehensive Guidance on How to Create a Yoga Program for Survivors

*Until we understand that traumatic symptoms are physiological as well as psychological, we will be woefully inadequate in our attempts to help them heal.*
—PETER LEVINE, *WAKING THE TIGER: HEALING TRAUMA*

There have been so many moments, books I have read, and trainings that I have attended that left me incredibly inspired and motivated and then I immediately asked myself: "But how am I actually going to make this a reality?!" The self-doubt and imposter syndrome have a way of creeping in, and sometimes we need extra support in making the transition from theory to practice. It felt important to me to share guidance on some starting points for how you might implement a trauma-informed yoga program in collaboration with a university or trauma agency or, if you are not a yoga teacher, how to infuse elements of this modality into the scope of your particular profession. Please keep in mind that each component of a full program implementation requires intentionality and thoughtfulness, and should be in collaboration within the framework of an established mental-health provider. This chapter will cover the following frameworks for creating and implementing a trauma-informed yoga program: (1) creating buy-in from a university/agency, (2) presenting powerful visuals and communicating your message, (3) using the power of collaborations, (4) working with mental health professionals, (5) identifying your niche and creating an intake process, (6) building a curriculum, (7) marketing and outreach, (8) understanding assessment and liability, and (9) honoring your voice. Please note: If you are not working with a university or another established mental health agency or provider, it's important to realize that when you start to incorporate work with trauma survivors, you may be dealing with confidential health information, which implicates the federal HIPAA law and state laws. So, you will have to consider additional or expanded confidentiality precautions and procedures, from vetted confidentiality forms to possibly HIPAA-compliant videoconferencing systems. Again, though, I strongly recommend that you work with an established mental-health agency or provider, who will have experience with this and will have protocols in place.

This is a critical and exciting time to be immersed in the field of trauma-informed yoga. People are listening, engaged, and invested. Now more than ever, administrators across the board—at universities, trauma agencies, and medical (and many other) settings—are passionate about expanding the scope of their services to be more holistic in nature. Leaving the body out of the healing process is no longer an option. And what a gift it is to provide survivors with a supportive pathway to reclaiming their own power, agency, and control.

I fully recognize how overwhelming it can feel to identify the best starting points for sharing your passion for this work. And remember, just as with the process of healing, this will take time. Please practice compassion with yourself as you create your own unique road map to doing this work. Your starting points might even begin with leading a trauma-informed savasana in the current yoga classes you are teaching; journaling empowering language and cues; integrating some of the tools, practices, or affirmations outlined in Chapter 6 into your clinical practice with clients; and/or making a list of community contacts who serve survivors of sexual assault and who you could potentially partner with. Start small and begin where you are. The frameworks below have taken me over 10 years to cultivate and it has been one incredible, heart-opening journey filled with tears, joy, rejection, success, and a lot of falling and getting back up again. Believe in yourself. I never imagined the curriculum that flowed from my own lived experience onto that piece of paper would be implemented so widely across the country. This is your reminder that you are absolutely capable of doing this work in ways that are sustainable and empowering and that fill you with joy. Remember when we talked about post-traumatic growth? This is absolutely part of that process. When we give ourselves the space to integrate the light and the dark, it helps us honor something my colleague Hala Khouri says, that "our gifts come from our wounds." Trust in your gifts and the power of your unique voice.

As you begin to identify your starting points, continue to build your program in ways that feel manageable and energizing to you. You can revisit my advice and guidance in small, digestible ways. You can pick and choose what resonates most with you. And most importantly, know that you are part of a larger trauma-informed community that is cheering you on, is engaged in this lifelong work with you, honors your passion, and knows how important this work is in the world.

## 1. How to Create Buy-In From a University or Agency

- **Create specific marketing materials that highlight the trauma-informed approach at its intersection with yoga.**
  - This might be creating flyers, business cards, a website, social media pages, or even your own press kit with all of this packaged together. What I have found is that the more specific I have been in my approach (i.e., working with sexual assault survivors), the easier it has been for me to narrow in on what my community networks might look like; they may include rape crisis centers, domestic-violence shelters, trauma agencies, sexual assault response offices, and counseling centers at universities. If it feels right for you, I encourage you to make

a list of the populations you feel passionate about serving and for which you have particular training, so you can carve out a niche or specialization to focus your efforts on.

- **Create a one-pager on trauma-informed yoga that includes research and tangible program benefits.**
  - I have provided you with a list of a number of research articles in the appendix that highlight trauma-informed yoga as an evidence-based modality for trauma survivors. Within your press kit or marketing materials, you might consider including a one-pager that outlines what the research demonstrates. Many academic environments and clinical settings will want to have an understanding of the science behind your program.

- **Draft an email highlighting your teaching background and introducing yourself and your program to the university/ agency. You could also consider this an opportunity to set up an in-person meeting with the staff person who is responsible for new programs or client services.**
  - Spend some time crafting an outreach email to introduce yourself to the centers that you would like to collaborate with. I have found that it is helpful to try to connect with the person who is responsible for survivor programs, as they will have the most oversight of a new program or the introduction of a new modality into their services. This would be an important time to discuss the need for modalities in addition to cognitive therapy and to have a conversation around the critical need for survivors to have multiple pathways to healing. You can review Chapters 1 and 2 for a refresher on talking points you might consider integrating.

- **Offer to do a free preview and short presentation on trauma-informed yoga for professional staff.**
  - After meeting with the main point of contact for new programs, you might offer to come to a staff meeting to provide a presentation on trauma-informed yoga. During this

presentation, consider leading a short practice or sharing specific tools so staff have an opportunity to feel the impact of the practice on their own bodies. Not only does this give them more of an understanding of how this program might land for their own clients, it also gives them an opportunity to practice self-care and even tend to their own experiences of compassion fatigue or burnout. The more allies you have on staff who want to see your program move forward, the better!

- **Propose a pilot program and conduct a thorough assessment.**
  - You could propose doing a pilot program (that you will still be paid to facilitate) but you could couple it with a thorough program assessment. I will share more on different ways to assess your program later in this chapter. When you can demonstrate the long-term impact of the program, you create more opportunities to make it sustainable. Additionally, it is so important to view this as a long-term modality as opposed to a one-time offering. We want to do our best to ensure that survivors can access trauma-informed yoga as an ongoing modality that is an integral part of trauma treatment.
- I will never forget when one of the first universities I consulted for added trauma-informed yoga to the list of their services on their brochure and website, and added it to their overall healing framework in the context of their outreach presentations. It might seem small, but it felt monumental in my heart. For years I had been working tirelessly to share my vision for sexual assault services to be more holistic in nature. We were suddenly reaching hundreds of survivors who found a healing modality that felt accessible to them.
- **Be up to date with current events at the university/agency.**
  - In the same way you might prepare for a job interview, you will want to do your due diligence in researching the university or agency where you hope to pitch your program. For

example, if there have been any recent Office of Civil Rights investigations or major Title IX complaints, it would be good to have a sense of the climate of the campus. This may offer context on potential barriers and on how you could address those concerns prior to meeting with staff. You will also want to research the services and programs that are currently being offered. Do they have other holistic offerings? How might trauma-informed yoga complement them or fill in gaps?

- **Build a proposal.**
  - In addition to teaching a trauma-informed yoga class for survivors, you may also want to support the university/ agency with building an intake process to assess a survivor's readiness for participation, provide guidance on assessment measures, and build a curriculum, among many other program elements. I encourage you to outline all of your offerings related to your program. The more integrated and comprehensive, the more easily it can be implemented into an organization that has the infrastructure to support it. And honestly, as a programmer myself for years in the anti-sexual violence field, I can say that the hardest part was having the time to create new content. Many staff at trauma agencies and in sexual-violence response centers on college campuses are inundated in the day-to-day work, seeing clients back-to-back, and responding to presentation and outreach requests. The more aspects of the content and implementation that you have identified ahead of time, the more supportive and easeful for everyone involved!

## 2. Present Powerful Visuals and Intentionally Communicate Your Message

I'll never forget when, a few years ago, I was asked to speak for 10 minutes on the agenda at the University of California (UC) President's Sexual Violence Task Force Meeting to discuss why trauma-informed yoga should be implemented as a modality at every UC campus. The room was composed of chiefs of police, Title IX directors, University of California regents, Campus Assault Resource and Education (CARE) staff, students . . . no pressure! I'm not sure of a time I felt more nervous. The presentation went well and this led to an amazing team who helped train yoga teachers and staff across each of the campuses in the trauma-informed modality and program implementation. I share this story to remind you that if you have only a few minutes to communicate your message and your passion for trauma-informed yoga for survivors, be intentional with your time and with how you communicate your message. During that presentation, each person received a handout that had a photo of the setup of the trauma-informed classes, a graph of the window of tolerance, clearly bolded charts that outlined the principles of trauma-informed yoga, anonymized survivor testimonials, summaries of program research and outcomes, and a description of the overall impact of the program. When I have facilitated PowerPoint presentations on this modality at a university/agency staff meeting, I have typically included the following:

- Visual of the somatic/physiological impact of trauma on the body
- A graph demonstrating an integrative and holistic approach to services
- An image of the window of tolerance to demonstrate how trauma-informed yoga is one modality to support survivors in widening their window and increasing their capacity for resilience
- Anonymized survivors' testimonials and research outcomes

Be creative and attuned to who your audience is so you can speak their language and highlight what is most relevant to them in the scope of their position. For example, when I speak to mental health professionals it feels important for me to connect with them on the ways in which our bodies hold trauma and on how trauma-informed yoga can complement the work that is happening in therapy. When I speak to law enforcement, I feel passionate about speaking to them about the neurobiology of trauma and why it is so challenging for survivors to recall specific details in a linear account about the trauma they have experienced. Additionally, they can better understand the context of my work when we have a conversation about how essential it is for survivors to find safety and stability in their nervous systems amid all of the barriers they encounter during the reporting and help-seeking process. Having a sense of who your audience is can help you tailor your presentation accordingly. Sometimes one powerful statement can speak right to someone's heart. And this can be the catalyst for seeing your program come to fruition.

## 3. Using the Power of Collaborations

I am a firm believer in collaborations of all kinds to make your program implementation a success. You were never meant to do this work alone or in isolation. Just as in the process of healing, your community is here to support you.

If you are currently teaching at a yoga studio, you might propose the idea of offering a weekly trauma-informed class to build interest and create a no-pressure drop-in class that survivors can attend when they are ready. When I taught a community trauma-informed yoga class at a donation-based studio, it became a well-utilized referral resource for local trauma therapists and a supportive place for survivors to find support and community. This is also a wonderful option for survivors who might not be ready to commit to a closed, 8-week class series. If you are worried about the stigma associated with having the term "trauma" listed in a class title, you could be creative with the name (e.g., Yoga for Self-Compassion, Yoga for Healing). In the description you could provide more detail regarding the trauma-informed framework that informs the class. Below is an example of how I describe my community class:

*Survivors of trauma, in the broadest definition of the word, share the experience of navigating their lives in the aftermath of a life-changing event(s). Survivors may have a range of body-based symptoms that pervade their entire lives, long after the trauma occurred. Bodily sensations associated with trauma can overwhelm the nervous system, which can create a lack of safety. Trauma permeates all aspects of one's lived experience: physical, psychological, mental, behavioral, social, and spiritual. Trauma-informed yoga and mindfulness practices offer modalities to help heal the whole person.*

*This class is designed to empower students to release trapped psychological and physical energies and come back home to their bodies. This gentle, trauma-informed meditation is coupled with light movement and supports students to feel more grounded and balanced, while focusing on natural breathing to promote relaxation, mindfulness, and embodiment.*

*Students are invited to channel quiet awareness and presence, find stability and safety in the body, and cultivate resilience. The postures and breath work are thoughtfully crafted to help uncover trauma imprints, support the healing process, create optimal balance of the nervous system, and lessen the grip that past experiences of trauma may have on the heart.*

## SPACE CONSIDERATIONS

If you collaborate with a local university or rape crisis center, you may find that they already have space available on-site, which is incredibly helpful when first building your program to help keep costs to a minimum. There are some additional benefits to working with an agency or university counseling center or sexual assault prevention and response center, including:

- An intake process is already established.
- Therapeutic implications are clear so each individual has a defined role (i.e., survivor advocate conducts intake process,

*(list continued on next page)*

*(list continued from previous page)*

trauma-informed yoga teacher leads class, clear discussions around consent and how information is shared).

- Liability and insurance are covered.
- There is an embedded structure for conducting research (if working with an academic institution).
- Financial structure is already established.
- Trauma-informed and culturally competent infrastructure is in place that supports the practice of yoga as an integral component of trauma treatment.

### FORM A COMMITTEE AND BUILD YOUR NETWORK

One of the most successful program implementations I had the honor of supporting was at a local university in California. They formed an entire committee of various staff from a cross section of student affairs departments. It can be very easy and exciting to get swept up in wanting to implement a program of this nature very quickly. But it is critical to think about systems and sustainability from the beginning and put processes in place to ensure that no single person is overwhelmed with all elements of the program. I have seen this occur a few times and those campuses or agencies struggled with long-term facilitation of the program because they didn't have proper processes or adequate staffing.

At the university I mentioned, there was a designated person in their student health center who conducted all of the survivor intakes; a trained trauma-informed yoga instructor who worked in their recreation center on campus; a well-thought-out referral process from the clinicians in their counseling center who specialized in working with survivors of sexual and intimate-partner violence; and a student staff team that helped with many programmatic elements, including marketing and helping the instructor with setup each week. The most important takeaway was that the committee worked collaboratively and shared the load of the program implementation. And each person was passionate about and invested in the program, which is why staff training to provide a foundation is so critical. As a result they had an incredible amount of interest from their survivor community and created a well-thought-out model that is now an integral support service as opposed to a one-time offering.

Lastly, you might also consider reaching out to your community of trauma-informed professionals who also work in the realm of Indigenous practices and holistic healing (meditation teachers, drum circle facilitators, art teachers, etc.). It can feel incredibly supportive to cofacilitate with additional practitioners and also introduce survivors to other healing modalities they can explore. And one of the gifts of cofacilitating? **You get to give and receive. You don't have to hold the container all on your own.**

## 4. Integrating Trauma-Informed Yoga Into Clinical Settings and Collaborating With Mental Health Professionals

Mental health professionals often reach out to me and ask if they need to attend a 200-hour yoga teacher training in order to integrate these tools into their clinical practice. I do feel that while having a strong understanding and foundation of yogic philosophy is important, there are still a number of tools that can be integrated within a therapeutic scope of practice.

### STARTING POINTS FOR INTEGRATING THIS MODALITY INTO CLINICAL PRACTICE

A common theme that mental health professionals share with me after integrating trauma-informed yoga into their work with clients is how often it creates a pathway for clients to be more expressive in therapy. We've discussed at length the ways in which the practice supports survivors in activating their parasympathetic nervous system, strengthening their vagal tone, widening their window of tolerance, and ultimately creating more space for safety, rest, and joy. When integrating these modalities, we send a powerful reminder to survivors: **They have always been worthy of a resilient nervous system.**

By taking a more holistic approach, we honor the way that trauma impacts a survivor's physical, social, emotional, and/or spiritual well-being. I am acutely aware of the moving work that happens within the walls of a therapist's office. Therapy has been a soft place to fall and a place to hold me in the depths of my despair. *Trigger/content warning related to pregnancy loss and trauma.* In 2016, I lost my son when I was 26 weeks pregnant. I will never forget the way the nurse held my hand and, through tears, told me that his heart was no longer beating. All of this was compounded by my ongoing healing from sexual trauma.

There were many times after the loss of my son that I came into therapy in a frozen state of grief and hypoarousal. My trauma symptoms would often flood my nervous system, and I spent my time filling in the space with work, distraction, and numbing so I didn't have to feel. It was much easier to escape my body than be present with my emotions, and that became a coping mechanism that I relied on. Talking about those physiological symptoms, although helpful, was not enough to thaw my grief. Taking the time to explore a few deep breaths at my pace, noticing what my feet felt like on the ground, and moving through some seated sun salutations could actually elevate my mood and help widen my window of tolerance. And to have the tools in therapy that allowed me to be even slightly more embodied, present, grounded, and safe helped create a pathway for more effective healing to take place. The subtle shifts of embodiment that accumulated over time have had the most meaningful long-term impact.

Below are some tangible tools that you might consider integrating into your clinical practice through a trauma-informed lens. *Please note, survivors may also find this section helpful, as it includes specific practices to support healing:*

- **Titration**
  - This refers to the process of slowing down the way we might jump into a new experience so we can work consciously with discomfort when it arises (Jo Buick, personal communication, October 13, 2019).
  - The first thing that comes to mind when I think about titration is the way we create space for all of our feelings exactly as they arise. When we begin to create space in a therapeutic

setting for the gift of embodiment, it can support survivors to be more resourced when they begin to engage with visceral reminders of their trauma histories, triggers, and survival skills.

- **Sadhana**
  - Sadhana is the Sanskrit word for daily spiritual practice. It is a daily yogic practice that connects you with your purpose.
  - Sadhana might refer to the restorative practices that survivors are weaving throughout their day to connect back to their intention or their healing. Spending some time in therapy discussing this concept and inviting survivors to brainstorm a list can support them in intentional choices around self-care. For example, the concept of daily Sadhana might be very helpful for a survivor who tends to practice self-care only after they have reached their breaking point. A daily Sadhana might be a tool to create more mindful awareness around how they tend to themselves in tiny pockets within their day. This might mean limiting phone time and overstimulation and replacing it with a walking meditation (bringing mindful attention to your experience without judgment), replacing trauma-related reading material with a light novel, giving themselves permission to take a nap in the middle of their day, or perhaps beginning their morning with journaling, a body scan, or gentle stretches in bed.

- **Sankalpa**
  - This is a Sanskrit word for intention or self-affirmation.
  - Beginning a therapy session with an intention can be a powerful way to guide the incredible collaborative work that is happening with the survivor. You might explore taking a few breaths together and invite them to rest a palm on heart and belly or find any gesture that feels comfortable to them. You could invite them to set an intention for your time together or to reflect upon what is resonating with them in that particular moment. After a few moments of breath and space, you might invite them to share what came up for them (if they would

like) and see how it guides the therapy session in an embodied way (Barnes & Crossley, personal communication, 2017).

- **Bhavana**
  - This is a Sanskrit word for visualization.
  - Exploring with visualization in a way that feels safe and accessible to the survivor can help to weave feelings of nourishment and ease into the therapy session. My own therapist ends each of our sessions with something called "calm place." I look forward to it every week because I know that amid really difficult conversations around boundaries or the painful triggers that arise when doing Eye Movement Desensitization and Reprocessing (EMDR), I will always have the opportunity for containment at the end of the session. She knows that being near the ocean, swimming with dolphins, walking on the sand, and sipping coffee are some of the most restorative images for me. You might explore working with your client to co-create what the "calm place" visualization looks like. Additionally, the ritual and routine of closing every session with it can be very stabilizing for your client's nervous system.
- **Meditation**
  - Meditation is a practice where an individual uses a technique—such as mindfulness, or focusing the mind on a particular object, thought, or activity—**to draw attention and awareness**, and work towards a mentally and emotionally calm state. You might explore incorporating trauma-informed meditation at the beginning or end of the therapy sessions. Feel free to visit the section on a trauma-sensitive approach to breath work and mindfulness in Chapter 3 for guidance around breath cues and language. My website and online course also include sample trauma-informed meditations, in addition to multiple lectures, to support you in implementing this work.
- **Grounding exercises**
  - **Grounding** creates calm, minimizes stress, and reminds us of who we are by diverting our attention from thinking and making us feel at home in our own bodies. Grounding exer-

cises are helpful to survivors not only as they navigate life in the aftermath of trauma but also amid difficult feelings that arise in the therapy session. This awareness provides them with tools to simultaneously tend to their inner landscape with gentleness and compassion. Below are just a few examples you might explore offering:

— Identify five things: you can see, you can hear, you can feel, you can taste, you can smell.
— Hold a grounding object.
— Rest palms on heart and belly.
— Notice your feet on the ground/notice what is supporting you in your chair.
— Integrate mindfulness into all aspects of the day (while in the therapy session, sipping coffee/tea, washing dishes, driving).
— Drink water.
— Take slow breaths at your pace.
— Self-hug.
— Journal.
— Cry.

- **Sensation**
  - During my trauma-sensitive yoga training with David Emerson and Jenn Turner, they shared how inviting students to connect to contrasts can support them with engaging with the present-moment experience. In my trauma-informed yoga classes I might invite a survivor to
    — notice the feeling of what is supporting them as they sit on their mat,
    — explore feeling the beat of their own heart,
    — notice the sound of their breath,
    — rub their palms together and create inner heat and maybe rest the palms over their heart to take in their own warmth,
    — rest a palm on their mat to feel the texture, or
    — hold a stone.
  - These are just a few tools you might invite survivors to explore to invite them back to the present when triggers

arise. When survivors continue to share details of their trauma and push through without any regard for the physiological messages of their bodies, it can end up causing more harm. When we engage the whole body and create space for and honor all of the feelings as they arise, **we remind survivors that all parts of them—mind, body, and spirit—are worthy of tending to.**

- ■ Movement
  - • I gave the example earlier about my own experience of moving through and shifting trauma residue when I was in an extreme state of hypoarousal during the most intense moments of my trauma and grief. Inviting survivors to move through seated or standing sun salutations, to explore neck rolls, or to find seated twists in their chair can support them with integrating movement into the therapy session. As always, you could present the survivor with a few choices and they could explore what resonates with them. You might also invite them to review the affirmations and postures in Chapter 6 (or in the trauma-informed yoga affirmation deck) and choose one that speaks to them in the moment. They may also feel empowered to couple a specific affirmation with their movement (for example, "I deserve to take up space" with Star Pose).
- ■ Affirmations
  - • You might revisit the survivor affirmations in Chapter 3 and integrate them into therapy sessions as it feels appropriate. You could invite the survivor you are working with to read them out loud or choose one at the end of each session that resonates with them or relates to a theme they explored in therapy that day.

## Mudra

*Mudra* is the Sanskrit word for "seal," "mark," or "gesture." Mudras are often used as hand gestures within contemplative practices to support healing and to send energy and support to different areas of the body.

Below are two of the mudras I frequently integrate into trauma-informed yoga classes; they can also be used as a tool in therapy to ground and honor a particular breakthrough or meaningful moment. They might also be incorporated as a way to support survivors with grounding or honoring their inner wisdom.

## Bhu Mudra

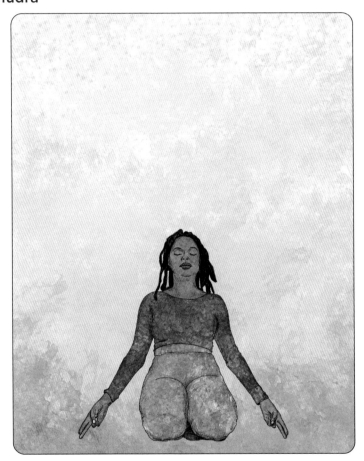

In Sanskrit, **Bhu** means "Earth" and **Mudra** means "gesture." One or both hands touch the ground. From a seated position, you might explore making peace fingers. If it feels right for you, you could explore grounding your peace fingers into the couch or chair or wherever you might be sitting at this moment. I invite you to connect with your breath in a way that feels accessible to you. Be gentle with yourself as you explore your breath and this sense of grounding and stability beneath you.

## Adi Mudra

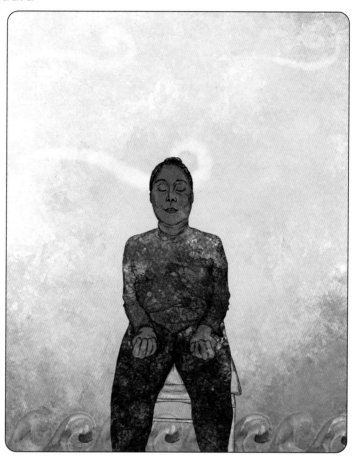

The Sanskrit term **Adi** means "first," and **Mudra** means "gesture." If you'd like you could explore bringing your thumbs into your palms and wrapping your fingers around your thumbs. You are always in choice around the degree and depth to which you'd like to squeeze your thumbs. Perhaps explore different levels of pressure to find what feels most comfortable for you. You could rest your palms on your knees facing up or down. Continue to explore your breath at your pace. You are worthy of finding moments of grounding amid the storm. Take your time. There is no rush.

Note: There are many moments throughout my day when I find that I am unconsciously practicing Adi Mudra. I will look down and realize the shape my palms make all on their own (almost as an innate and intuitive response to when I need to access safety or grounding). You never know how exploring with mudras might become a go-to tool for your body without much awareness!

> A NOTE ON LANGUAGE: I want to invite you to revisit the section on empowerment-based language in Chapter 3 before starting to implement some of these tools in your therapy practice. This ensures you feel comfortable sharing the tools in a way that puts the survivor at the center of their own experience and honors the pace in which they feel ready to engage with the tools. You might also consider small ways in which you can integrate choice into your sessions—asking students, for example, where they would like to sit in the room, how the temperature and lighting feel, if they would like to begin with an embodied practice, and so on.

Please also note that if you are a social-justice educator, facilitator, educator, coach, doula, faculty member, or any other professional who holds space for survivors, you can absolutely adapt some of these practices into your work! Explore your own variations and tailor them to your needs and scope of practice.

## YOGA TEACHER COLLABORATIONS WITH MENTAL HEALTH PROFESSIONALS

By working collaboratively with mental health professionals, we can provide a comprehensive approach to healing sexual trauma. In addition to the impact that trauma-informed yoga can have on helping survivors be more expressive in therapy, we have a valuable opportunity to train mental health professionals in trauma-informed yoga approaches to utilize in talk therapy with their clients. Below are a few examples of types of mental health professionals as outlined by the National Alliance on Mental Illness (NAMI, 2020):

- Psychologists
  - Doctor of Philosophy (PhD)
  - Doctor of Psychology (PsyD)
- Counselors, clinicians, therapists
  - Master's degree (MS or MA) in a mental health field: psychology, counseling psychology, marriage or family therapy, etc.
  - Licensed Professional Counselor (LPC)
  - Licensed Marriage and Family Therapist (LMFT)
  - Licensed Clinical Alcohol and Drug Abuse Counselor (LCADAC)
- Clinical social workers
  - Licensed Independent Social Worker (LICSW)
  - Licensed Clinical Social Worker (LCSW)
  - Academy of Certified Social Workers (ACSW)
- Psychiatrists
  - Doctor of Medicine (MD) or Doctor of Osteopathic Medicine (DO) and residency training in psychiatry
- Other:
  - Certified Peer Specialist
  - Social Worker
  - Pastoral Counselor

Below are bottom-up treatments for PTSD as outlined by Dr. Kristen Zaleski (personal communication, September 2, 2015) that may help to calm the nervous system and work well in conjunction with trauma-informed yoga. This is about first establishing safety with the survivor and introducing mindfulness before jumping into the trauma narrative.

- Breathing retraining
- Mindfulness meditation and other manualized treatments such as mindfulness-based stress reduction

- Somatic experiencing
- Sensorimotor psychotherapy
- EMDR

There are multiple program formats for collaborating with mental health professionals for you to consider. You may also determine this after meeting with a university/agency to better understand their infrastructure, liability and confidentiality policies, staffing, and needs. Below are some options to explore:

- Therapist helps with intake process and determining survivor readiness for the program.
- Cofacilitate the trauma-informed yoga series with a therapist who will be present for all classes and lead a psycho-educational component on other topics (self-care, assertiveness, boundaries, sleep, chronic stress, depression/anxiety, etc.).
- Collaborate with therapist to help provide direct support for students who might be triggered in class.
- Propose an integration of trauma-informed yoga with a sexual assault support group/group counseling.
- The Justice Resource Center recommends that clients who practice trauma-sensitive yoga also work with a therapist who has specialized training in trauma.
- Offer a training for mental health professionals on how to integrate trauma-informed yoga into their individual sessions with clients.

**Most importantly, develop a program format with clear guidelines for each facilitator so all parties feel comfortable.**

*When I facilitate the 8-week trauma-informed yoga program, I receive direct referrals from therapists and survivor advocates who are trained in appropriate referrals to the program. I do not require survivors to be in therapy. The reason for this is that many survivors start with the yoga program and then feel empowered to seek additional mental health resources (e.g., scheduling an appointment with a therapist or survivor advocate).*

## 5. Identifying Your Audience and Creating an Intake Process

If you are running a trauma-informed yoga group, class, or series at your university or trauma agency, it is important to develop an intake and screening process to assess a survivor's readiness for participation in the program. This allows you to support them holistically in the process of navigating resources and identifying the options that feel best for them.

### Eligibility

- Take the time to develop a screening and intake process, intake form, and waiver. Something I have found to be particularly powerful is creating a body-inclusive form and/or an emotion chart where survivors can share where they might be holding trauma in their bodies, current symptoms they may be experiencing, and injuries (if they feel comfortable). This allows you to integrate a trauma-informed framework even within the scope of your policies and forms, as it offers survivors different ways to express their emotions and their experiences of trauma.
- The Justice Resource Center recommends that potential participants who have had recent hospitalizations, have active drug and alcohol abuse, have experienced sexual victimization very recently, or have current psychosis not be recommended to participate.
- It is important to contain the safety of the room, and this process helps you work directly with the survivor to identify whether the program is the right fit at this point in their healing process. For example, if a survivor has experienced sexual victimization very recently, the recommendation may be to focus on safety and stability first and connect them with immediate safety resources and referrals (medical support,

advocacy, reporting, etc.) to access on their terms, when and if they feel ready.
- Be authentic and open with survivors about the process. It is important to set clear boundaries early on, kindly and empathetically.
- I recommend no more than 10–15 students in a closed-series format, especially in your initial stages of offering a group of this kind.
- A collaboration with a mental health professional may be the most effective way to pitch the program, as agencies may be apprehensive about implementing a program without that type of supervision.

*Once you have your forms ready and survivor referrals have come in, it is time for the survivor-intake process; see below for a step-by-step outline for conducting this:*

**Step 1, Intake Meeting:**
- To begin, identify the person on campus or at your organization who will conduct the intake process to identify survivor readiness for the program. This looks different for each organization, given the unique needs of each population and the resources available, but ideally this person would be a survivor advocate, clinician, or confidential employee with experience in working with trauma survivors.
- It is important to be open and clear with survivors about the intake process. This is the beginning of establishing clear boundaries with potential participants. Think about creating a trauma-informed and comfortable space where you can facilitate the intake meeting.
- Informed and thoughtful judgment is advised in determining readiness and recommendation for the program.
- The intake process also helps you to be thoughtful about addressing any safety concerns with the group.

**Step 2, Interest Form:**

- All of the details related to collection of forms will vary based on your site needs, confidentiality requirements, and general program structures (i.e., how students submit their interest forms, who receives them, who schedules the intake, etc.).

- Ensure that the waiver is signed. If the participant is a minor, it has to be signed by their parent or guardian.

- A symptom checklist gives facilitators an idea of the potential impact of trauma on the body and/or any special needs to be considered as the trauma-informed yoga teacher prepares the class series.

- A body-inclusive form allows clients to focus on areas where there are injuries or areas of the body that may hold their trauma. Additionally, this form can help the instructor curate a trauma-informed yoga practice that attends to symptom trends, physical complaints, and so on. If the instructor leading the training has attended a Transcending Sexual Trauma Through Yoga 3-day in-person or online training, they will receive more training regarding this process.

**Step 3, Documentation:**

- **Create a plan with the survivor.** This may entail asking for a release of information, to discuss the following with the yoga instructor: trauma symptoms, safety concerns, or injuries a student may have.

- **Create a plan for documentation/storage of interest forms.** If you are offering a closed group for survivors, discuss with your staff how you will document yoga notes, store records, and store HIPAA sensitive information, within the framework of the organization you're working with.

- **Writing a yoga note.** If you are in a dual role as a therapist and yoga instructor, you might consider integrating yoga notes into your clinical practice to demonstrate the impact of working holistically with a survivor in their treatment goals. The note below is an example from Dr. Shena Young (personal communication, January 30, 2017). This may be more clinical than you need, but it may be helpful for you to see an example of what this looks like should you choose to incorporate this process into your program.

*The theme of the session was creating safety. Group members were reintroduced to one another, asked to complete baseline evaluations, invited to share their decorated safety jars, and engaged in a discussion about Chapters 1 and 2 in the* Emotional Yoga *book. Group concluded with a 45-minute trauma-informed yoga practice and completion of a post-practice evaluation. They were encouraged to read Chapter 3 for next week and to practice the concept of allowance.*

*Tati was engaged and reflective throughout. She was observed to be timid in sharing her thoughts but successful in communicating plans for self-care practices in the next week. She was also observed to make choices during the yoga practice as she experimented with pace, choice, and posture variations.*

- **Release of information.** There have been many cases where I have had a release of information from the survivor's therapist and it has been a wonderful, integrative, and collaborative approach to supporting the survivor. For example, if there were certain breakthroughs happening during trauma-informed yoga around choice or boundary setting, I could speak with the therapist and they could build upon that work in session. I saw some of the most profound healing happen through this collaboration. Find what works best for your program and continue to try out different elements until you find the best fit!

## 6. Building a Curriculum

At the beginning of the book I shared a bit about my process of developing the 8-week survivor curriculum. The best advice I can give is to write a curriculum from your heart. I have found that survivors deeply appreciate a curriculum and a program that resonate with their lived experience and allow them to feel seen and heard. Below gives you an overview and the structure and scope of my curriculum (© Zahabiyah Yamasaki). My sincere hope is that I can be a compassionate conduit and that it inspires you in the creation and development of your own. I can't wait to see all you will create and all the lives you will impact through your voice and your gifts.

### CLASS STRUCTURE AND ACTIVITIES

The 8-week trauma-informed yoga series offers survivors an empowering space to gain greater awareness around various concepts and anchors, including inner strength, safety, boundaries, and assertiveness, among many others. Classes focus on restorative and vinyasa postures, support the nervous system, explore positive affirmations, and are also coupled with guided activities, including debriefing exercises, meditation, journaling, art, and drumming. Classes support survivors in reconnecting with themselves and building community with their peers.

Each class is typically 90 minutes:

**First 30 minutes:**
- Includes brief discussion of theme
- Includes activity related to the weekly theme; a few examples include:
  - **Intention stones**
    - Each class, survivors are given a stone and a metallic marker and invited to write their intention for class. This becomes a tangible reminder of what they hope to cultivate each week.
  - **Surrender bowl**
    - This activity involves passing out small sheets of dissolvable paper or index cards to each survivor and placing a

medium-sized bowl of water in the center of the circle of yoga mats. I typically start the first class of the 8-week series with this activity, to invite the participating survivors to release something that does not serve them. They are invited to release the paper into the bowl—a symbolic gesture for releasing it and creating more space.

- **Take-what-you-need board**
  - This activity involves a large white poster board that has multiple Post-it Notes on it with various words, including "healing," "rest," "joy," "community," "energy," "time," "strength," and so on. Survivors are invited during each class to "take what they need," and place the Post-it somewhere visible as a daily reminder to take steps to cultivate what they need more of in their lives.
- **Safety jars**
  - This activity includes passing out mason jars to each participant to cultivate safety and self-care. Toward the beginning of the series, survivors are invited to decorate the jars with items that make them feel nourished or whole or remind them of positive experiences of healing, photos of people that are important to them, quotes, affirmations, and/or photos of places that bring them calm and peace. The safety jar becomes a container for their intention stones and a tangible reminder of all of the incredible work they have dedicated to their healing process.
  - I will never forget a story that one survivor shared with me about her safety jar. After navigating much turmoil around self-worth and challenging relationships, she found her life partner within some significant healing. Her partner suggested that they place her safety jar as a centerpiece on their sweetheart table at their wedding as a reminder of her resilience and the strength of their love. You never know the ways these tools will inspire the lives of survivors you work with. This story brings me to tears every single time.

- **Self-care wheel**
  - Olga Phoenix (2015) has developed a wonderful self-care wheel that focuses on various dimensions of well-being, including physical, psychological, emotional, spiritual, personal, and professional. It may be helpful to invite survivors to review the different categories and then also invite them to fill out a blank wheel to personalize their self-care plan. I try to encourage survivors to pick just one thing to focus on in each category so self-care does not become another overwhelming aspect of their lives.
- **Letters to self**
  - This is a powerful writing exercise that invites students to write a letter to themselves about the goals they have for the program and their own healing journey. I include paper and an envelope in their workbooks and they seal it and give it back to me whenever they are ready. I pass the letters back out on week 8 of the program to give them a chance to reflect on how far they've come. It is beautiful to witness their often tearful yet joyful reactions.

**Next 60 minutes:**
- The next half of class includes the facilitation of a trauma-informed yoga class centered around the following variation of themes:
  - Week 1
    - *Theme: Orientation and Intention*
    - *Mantra: I am held and supported in my healing journey.*
  - Week 2
    - *Theme: Safety*
    - *Mantra: I am safe, I am loved, I am home, I am in my body.*
  - Week 3
    - *Theme: Self-Care as a Daily Practice*

- *Mantra: I am enough just as I am. I allow myself to rest. My productivity does not determine my worth. I am doing my best. That is enough.*
  - Week 4
    - *Theme: Embodied Boundaries*
    - *Mantra: My boundaries support me with honoring my truth. I release what does not serve me. I reclaim more space for me.*
  - Week 5
    - *Theme: Assertiveness*
    - *Mantra: I am courageous, I am fearless, I am inherently whole. I honor my value and my power.*
  - Week 6
    - *Theme: Self-Compassion*
    - *Mantra: I remind myself that I am worthy of my own energy, time, and affection.*
  - Week 7
    - *Theme: Inner Strength and Trust*
    - *Mantra: I am not defined by the darkness I have experienced. I honor the power of my resilience and my light. I trust the strength of my body to hold me today.*
  - Week 8
    - *Theme: Cultivating Community*
    - *Mantra: I feel the support of my community. I feel grounded, confident, worthy, and whole. I am not alone in my experience.*

**Supplemental classes in the series might also include:**
- **Art as Healing**
  - During week 6 we work with an amazing artist, Eve Andry (illustrator of the yoga postures in this book), who creates custom canvas mat covers so survivors can paint on the safety and support of their mats. She integrates various prompts for them to express their inner world and feelings

onto a canvas. This class always makes me think of the Georgia O'Keeffe quote: "I found I could say things with color and shapes that I couldn't say any other way—things I had no words for." I find this to be one of the most powerful classes in the series, as it invites students to express themselves in an entirely new way.

- **Drumming**
  - We close our final class of the 8-week series with a drum circle with an organization called HealthRHYTHMS. Instead of asking survivors to share what the past 8 weeks have been like for them, the facilitator invites them to play it on the drum. There is one story that has stayed with me all these years. There was a survivor who enrolled in the program and was initially very apprehensive. She typically preferred not to share or connect with the group. But week after week, you saw her slowly pulling down her emotional layers at a pace that felt comfortable and safe for her. She started sharing with the other participants, smiling, and engaging during activities. She was the first person to ask if she could play on the drum what the experience in the program was like for her. She began with a very slow and light drum beat and then it sped up and became very fast and loud. If the survivor is comfortable, we ask if we can share back what we thought we heard. I shared this with her: "I felt that when you began the program you were apprehensive and struggled with trust. But each week we all witnessed your beautiful healing unfold. We saw you step into your power and truth, and who you have always been, but that person got covered up a bit because of your experiences with trauma. We got to see you bloom." She shared through tears that this was exactly what the experience was like for her.

However you design and develop your own curriculum will be wonderful and unique to your gifts, your lived experience, and the communities you work with. I hope the examples above provide hope and inspiration for all that is possible. Give yourself permission to start small and go slowly. Take all the time you need to tend to the needs of your own nervous system before putting too much pressure on yourself to create something.

## 7. Marketing and Outreach

There are many different ways to consider the marketing and outreach of your trauma-informed yoga classes. I also recognize this will vary depending on whether you are teaching at a specific agency/university or marketing your own classes—both are incredible services to the community.

If you are working with an agency/university to offer this modality as a part of their services, I encourage you to meet with the survivor advocates, clinicians, and staff to explain the intake process so they can make direct referrals to the program. If you are marketing a drop-in trauma-informed yoga class that you are offering in the community or at a studio space, you might consider the following:

- Build a website that highlights your trauma-informed approach.
- Create a flyer that highlights your classes that you can share with trauma therapists in your area, on social media, and with local universities and trauma agencies. Some of my favorite resources for making flyers are:
  - Canva: https://www.canva.com
  - Fiverr: https://www.fiverr.com
  - Unsplash: https://unsplash.com
- Please note: Be sure to read the terms of use of any site whose resources you use, so that you know exactly what you are allowed to do with those materials on your site, and so that, in the case of a site that offers free photos, you understand any legal risks of using those photos.
- You may want to create social media pages and highlight survivor testimonials to show the impact of your work (but

you must obtain clear and unequivocal consent to that exact use from the survivors whose testimonials you want to use and you must anonymize the material, not just by changing or omitting names and initials, but by omitting any details of their experience that would make it possible for others to identify them).

- Send personal emails to local domestic-violence shelters, rape crisis centers, and sexual assault response offices.
- Spend some time networking with local therapists or private practices that specialize in trauma-informed care and that work with survivors of sexual trauma. Perhaps drop off a stack of flyers they can easily share with clients.
- Ask your yoga studio if they could do a teacher profile on your trauma-informed yoga class and add it to their newsletter or highlight it on social media channels.
- Offer to facilitate compassion-fatigue classes for staff at the agencies/universities where you are pitching your program. This gives them the gift of self-care and may also inspire them to attend your classes in the community.
- Personalized and multiple approaches are key!

## 8. Understanding Assessment and Liability

Assessment and evaluation of our programs is typically the last thing we prioritize, but it should be the first. Ongoing program assessment is critical, especially when beginning with first-time or pilot programs. Any form of evaluation-even a brief pre and post test- allows you to understand how the program is impacting survivors, to think about changes that need to be made in response to their feedback, and to build a foundation for the program to be sustainable.

Below are some general points of reference to keep in mind as you begin to build your assessment process:

## IDENTIFY PROGRAM GOALS

I invite you to spend some time in thoughtful reflection regarding the goals for your trauma-informed yoga program. Below are some preliminary goals I developed when I began my very first program:

GOAL 1: *Help survivor participants develop positive coping mechanisms.*

GOAL 2: *Help survivor participants feel empowered to seek additional support services.*

GOAL 3: *Help survivor participants build a community of support.*

This process will be unique to each individual, but if you need ideas, you might refer back to the list of trauma-informed yoga program benefits outlined in Chapter 1. This gives you a sense of the impact that the practice has had on the healing process for survivors and may give you some inspiration as you conceptualize your assessment and identify questions that feel aligned.

## DEVELOP QUESTIONS TO ASSESS PROGRAM GOALS

If you are putting together a pre- and post-test, take time to review your program goals and develop a list of questions to assess those overarching goals. Always include language for survivors to opt out of any questions that do not feel comfortable, opt out of the assessment altogether, and/or answer questions anonymously. Sample questions might include:

1. I invite you to rate the effectiveness of the tools you currently have to assist you in managing triggers.
2. I invite you to rate the effectiveness of any additional modes of healing you have utilized to aid you in your healing process.
3. I invite you to rate the degree you currently feel safe in your body.
4. I invite you to rate the effectiveness of your current support system.

For those who might be offering programs within an academic setting, there may be meaningful opportunities for collaboration with faculty, graduate students, and researchers to conduct something more comprehensive with Institutional Review Board (IRB) approval.

## OTHER ASSESSMENT MEASURES

Below are a few additional ideas to infuse assessment and collection of feedback throughout your trauma-informed yoga program:

---

**Validated scales to explore referencing to assess your program:**

- Beck Anxiety Inventory (BAI)
- Center for Epidemiologic Studies Depression Scale (CES-D)
- Coping Strategies Scale
- Impact of Event Scale (IES)
- Mindful Attention Awareness Scale (MAAS)
- Posttraumatic Stress Disorder Checklist (PCL)
- Self-Compassion Scale (SCS)
- Scale of Body Connection (SBC)

---

I had the honor of working with eight campuses in California that implemented the 8-week trauma-informed yoga program curriculum. We worked with Meghan Davidson, PhD, a researcher from the University of Nebraska who secured IRB approval to conduct the research. She worked with the campuses to measure the following:

---

- psychological symptoms: depression, anxiety, PTSD
- self-compassion: mindfulness, self-kindness, self-judgment, common humanity, isolation
- body awareness and dissociation
- safety

---

At the onset of this process, I was tasked with training the identified yoga teachers across each California campus on how to teach from a trauma-informed lens. A number of teachers who were already facilitating the curriculum then trained the staff at each sexual assault response office.

The assessment process as outlined by the researcher involved a pre-test, a post-test, and an 8-week follow-up. The sexual assault response offices provided an informed-consent process and online questionnaire during the survivor-intake process, as well as attendance sheets and checklists to confirm the facilitation of the curriculum (to ensure some sense of consistency across each campus). And lastly, students were invited to fill out the same online questionnaire at the end of the last session of the 8-week series, and again 8 weeks later.

The outcomes of this study demonstrated significant decreases in depression, anxiety, PTSD symptoms, self-judgment, dissociation, and isolation. We saw significant increases in self-compassion, body awareness, and mindfulness (Davidson, 2019). Survivors have known this to be true in their bodies for years, but for me to be able to formally say that this curriculum is evidence-based has been an amazing feat and journey.

## 9. Honoring Your Voice, Connecting to Joy, and Self-Compassion as an Ongoing Practice

*Take note of shifts in your energy and your nervous system when you are around people and places that honor your boundaries and celebrate your rest. You are worthy of safety and ease.*

While I hope this chapter has provided you with a strong foundation on which to build upon your gifts, I want to remind you to always trust and honor your own voice. Grounding yourself in your truth and your unique journey will inspire you to do the work from a place of authenticity and love. Those are the most critical qualities in moving this work forward—in your own ways and at your own pace. Take the time to sit with your intentions, to honor your capacity, to identify the populations you are passionate about working with, and to allow things to unfold on their own timeline.

I want to invite you to take frequent moments in the midst of this journey to connect to what brings you joy. I have been trying to remind myself that joy is a piece of the fabric of sustainable activism. According to Isaias Hernandez, "sustainable activism" is defined as:

> Ways in which you find practices in your work that are everlasting, regenerative, and equitable. Implementing systems where you can ensure that you can "confidently engage in for years, not just weeks." It also advocates for your environment, community, and yourself to find ways of healing when fighting for justice. (@queerbrownvegan, Instagram, June 26, 2020)

I have been guilty of pushing myself beyond my capacity these days. With actively engaging in antiracism work, supporting survivors, mothering, and working full-time amid this pandemic—rest and joy have felt unattainable, as so many of us are in survival mode. One of the practices that continues to ground me in joy is **self-compassion**.

I think the greatest gift of self-compassion is that it comes in so many forms. Sometimes for me self-compassion means rest, boundaries, centering and grounding amid my advocacy work, closing my eyes instead of staring at my screen, self-love, connection, taking a deep breath before doing just about anything, pausing, reclaiming my time, not being so hard on myself, opting in, opting out, engaging in an activity that nourishes me or makes me smile, yoga, and everyday mindfulness.

We are so lucky to have so many resources accessible to us. And in the age of information and overstimulation, it is likely that our nervous systems are absorbing material all the time at an urgent pace. Our bodies were not designed to integrate trauma-related material this quickly, or do anything this quickly! If you are exhausted and fatigued, you are not alone. Pace yourself and your energy. Find ways to do the work sustainably. And prioritize moments of compassion, joy, and rest wherever possible. Sometimes finding small ways to integrate this work into our lives can help us manage the overwhelm of our lifelong work as trauma-informed practitioners.

Your work awaits you at a tender and compassionate pace. I cannot wait to see all the ways you will inspire survivors, build community, offer accessible healing, and quite literally save and change lives. I will be here cheering you on, while sending you frequent reminders to tend to your needs and care. And to reclaim rest as a radical practice. And in case you need the reminders:

You don't have to earn your rest.

You are worthy and enough, just as you are.

Your productivity does not determine your worth.

You are worthy when you are napping.

You are worthy when you say you are at capacity.

You are worthy when you need support.

You are worthy when you're struggling.

You are worthy of taking your time.

You are worthy of your care.

You are worthy when you don't have the bandwidth to support others.

You are worthy of being seen.

You are worthy of taking up space.

You are worthy of appreciation.

You are worthy when you breakdown.

You are worthy when you're overwhelmed.

You are worthy of your energy.

You are worthy of ease and space.

You are worthy of tending to your mental health.

You are worthy of grace.

You are worthy of compassion, support, affirmation, and understanding.

You are worthy of joy.

You are worthy of fun.

You are worthy of love.

Week and class theme:

Date:

Name or student ID number:

### Before Trauma-Informed Yoga Practice

I invite you to compassionately check in with yourself and take a scan of your body and your needs before the yoga practice. Everything below is an invitation. You are welcome to answer anything that feels comfortable to you.

**How is your heart?**

_____

_____

**How are you feeling physically?**

| 1 | 2 | 3 | 4 | 5 | 6 | 7 | 8 | 9 | 10 |
|---|---|---|---|---|---|---|---|---|---|
| Low | | | | Neutral | | | | | Well |

Notes:

_____

_____

**How are you feeling emotionally?**

| 1 | 2 | 3 | 4 | 5 | 6 | 7 | 8 | 9 | 10 |
|---|---|---|---|---|---|---|---|---|---|
| Low | | | | Neutral | | | | | Well |

Notes:

_____

_____

**Is there anything else you would like to share?**

_____

_____

Week and class theme:

Date:

Name or student ID number:

**After Trauma-Informed Yoga Practice**

I invite you to compassionately check in with yourself and take a scan of your body and your needs after the yoga practice. Everything below is an invitation. You are welcome to answer anything that feels comfortable to you.

How is your heart?

_____

_____


How are you feeling physically?

| 1 | 2 | 3 | 4 | 5 | 6 | 7 | 8 | 9 | 10 |
|---|---|---|---|---|---|---|---|---|----|
| Low | | | | Neutral | | | | | Well |

Notes:

_____

_____


How are you feeling emotionally?

| 1 | 2 | 3 | 4 | 5 | 6 | 7 | 8 | 9 | 10 |
|---|---|---|---|---|---|---|---|---|----|
| Low | | | | Neutral | | | | | Well |

Notes:

_____

_____

What is something you are taking with you from today's practice?

_____

_____

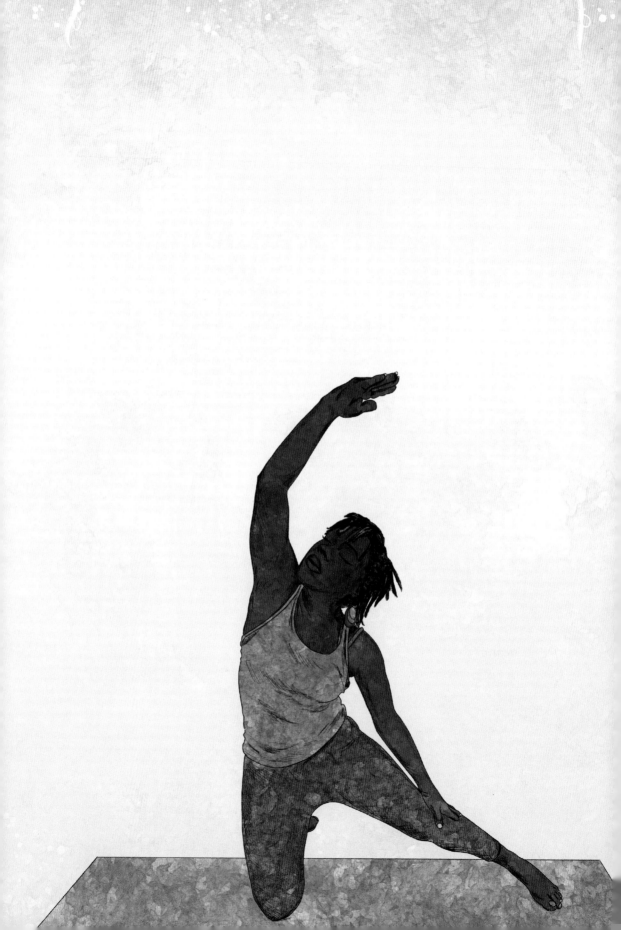

# · 6 ·

# Trauma-Informed Yoga Tool Kit and Affirmations

*You can be healed and still healing.*
*You can be open and still hurting.*
*You can be brave and still frightened.*

—REBECCA RAY,
EXCERPT FROM *THE UNIVERSE LISTENS TO BRAVE*

I hope you find this chapter to be a supportive place to learn affirmations that are coupled with trauma-informed yoga practices to explore integrating into your healing process. This chapter will also be an informative reference point for yoga instructors, mental health professionals, educators, and other healing professionals who are looking for guidance on practices and curricula to share with survivors in classes, workshops, or clinical practice.

## Setting Up Your Space

If you are cultivating an at-home practice, I invite you to spend some time setting up your space in a way that feels supportive, comfortable, and

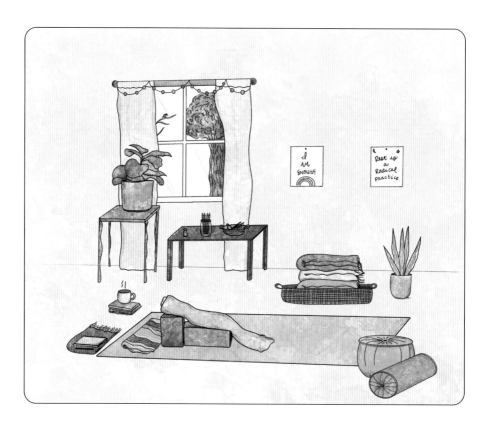

meaningful to you. You might explore creating an emotional-safety ritual (adapted from Davis, 1990), which is essentially an opportunity to carve out time in your day just for you. You may want to have a yoga mat and props, play music, or surround yourself with objects that you feel connected to. You may want to tidy up your space or have a cup of tea. It is an opportunity for you to create a consistent ritual to support stabilizing your nervous system and to have a dedicated space to tend to your needs that you can look forward to each day. It could be as short as 5 minutes or as long as several hours.

Your practice is a sacred opportunity to reconnect to yourself. You may choose to communicate with your family, roommates, friends, and community about your designated practice time so it can remain uninterrupted. As you start to prepare for your practice you might take some time to check in with yourself by taking a mindful body scan to assess your needs or perhaps by filling out the baseline card shown in the diagram. This gives you an opportunity to check in with how you are feeling before and after your practice. Sometimes it can also feel nice to see a tangible reminder of your progress.

## Journaling

- It may feel supportive to journal after your practice:
- Spend some time in reflection. What was your experience? What did you notice around choice and agency? What did you enjoy? What felt challenging? No need to judge anything about your experience. All of your feelings and emotions are valid. You are enough just as you are.
- Is there an intention you can write on your intention stone or an anchor you might bring with you as you move through the rest of your day?

## Trauma-Informed Yoga Tool Kit for Survivors

Below you will find a series of affirmations, postures, cues, and invitations. If you would like, you could even record the cues on your phone to support you when moving through the posture variations. As always, you are in choice around what feels best for your body. As you read through the affirmations, take note of how they land on your heart. If there is a different posture, expression, or movement that comes up for you—please listen to your body! You are the expert of you, and what you see below are gentle invitations. Take your time and move at your pace. The choices you make with your body are celebrated. There is absolutely no rush.

# BUTTERFLY POSE

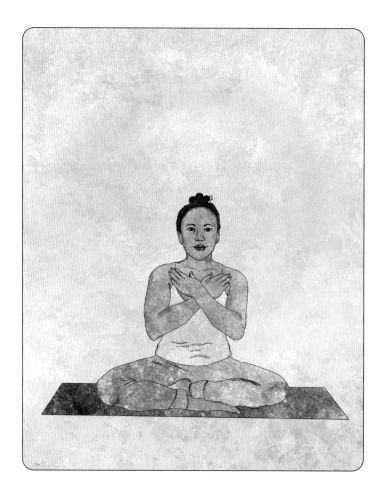

AFFIRMATION: I am not alone in this experience.

INVITATION: I invite you to find a comfortable seated posture. If it feels right, you could cross your arms across your chest. Perhaps rest the right side of your cheek on your left palm and offer yourself a gentle hug. If it feels safe to continue, please feel free to explore this motion side to side. I invite you to integrate a gentle rocking movement if that feels good for you. You are never alone in your experience.

# UTTHITA TADASANA

(STAR POSE)

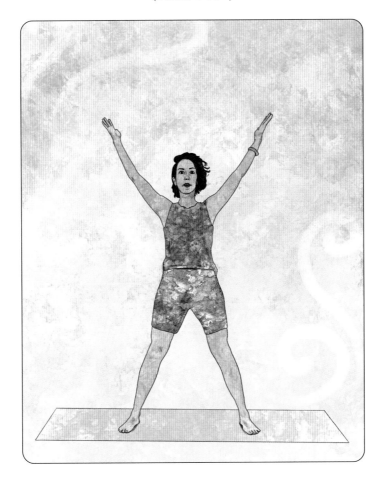

AFFIRMATION: I deserve to take up space.

INVITATION: From a standing posture, I invite you to bring your legs hip distance apart and extend your arms toward the sky. You might explore making a V shape with your arms. If you would like, you could take your gaze up toward the sky and repeat the affirmation: "I deserve to take up space." Please explore any variations of this posture that feel accessible and supportive in your body. All of you is welcome here.

# ANJANEYASANA

## (CRESCENT MOON)

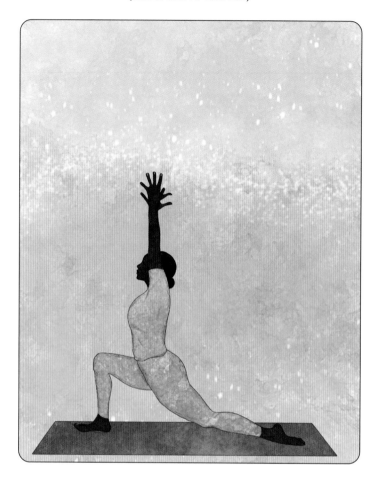

AFFIRMATION: I honor the layers of my diverse and unique lived experience.

INVITATION: If it feels okay, feel free to bend your front knee and bring your back knee to the ground. If you experience any tension in your knee, you could rest a blanket underneath your knee or roll up your mat to create an additional layer of support. On your inhale breath, you might explore extending your arms high to the sky. If it feels right in your body, bring your palms to a steeple grip, and invite your thumb and index finger to rest together. Notice the strength of your body. Honor all that you do and all that you hold.

# SUKHASANA
## (COMFORTABLE POSE)

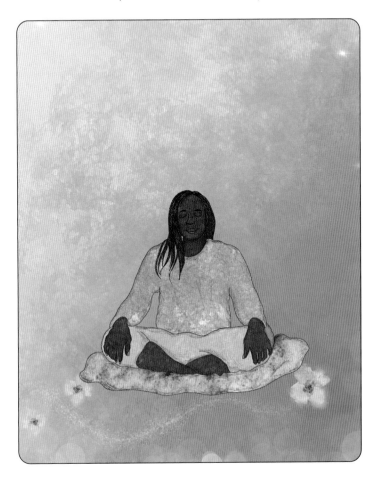

AFFIRMATION: I am healing, even when it's hard.

INVITATION: If you would like, you can begin in any form of seated that feels right for your body. Perhaps on a mat, bolster, or chair. You might explore bringing one hand to your belly and one hand to your heart. Take a moment to notice the rise and fall of your breath. I invite you to turn the volume of your heart all the way up, and the volume of your thoughts all the way down. This is your body and your practice. Take all the time you need here. There is no rush. Perhaps recite the affirmation: "I am healing, even when it's hard."

# BALASANA

(RESTORATIVE CHILD'S POSE)

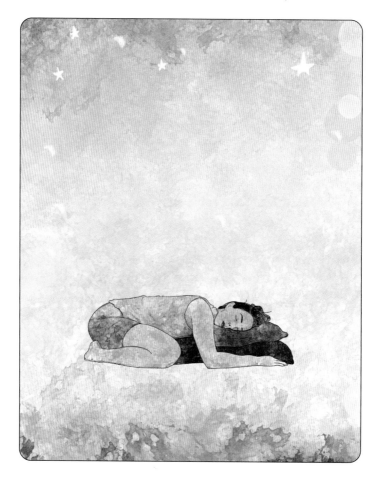

AFFIRMATION: I deserve to rest.

INVITATION: If you have a pillow, yoga bolster, or blanket nearby, and you'd like to integrate it into your practice, please feel free to reach for it. I invite you to rest your body over the prop and invite your knees to the outside edges of your mat, if that feels comfortable to you. You can make any adjustments with your arms that feel right, perhaps holding the prop or resting your arms by your sides. You can lay your cheek on the prop and rest here for as long as you need. I invite you to repeat and embody the affirmation: "I deserve to rest."

# TADASANA

(MOUNTAIN POSE)

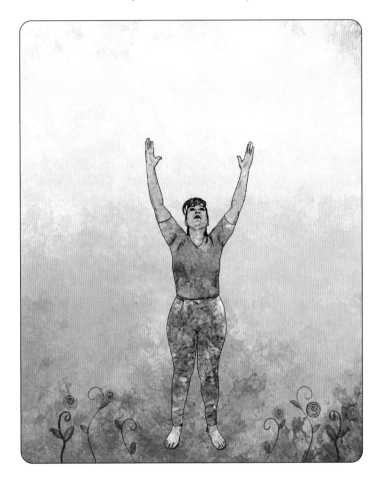

AFFIRMATION: I trust the strength of my body to hold me today.

INVITATION: From seated or standing, I invite you to explore bringing your feet hip distance apart. On your inhale, maybe extend your arms high to the sky—sending energy through your fingertips. You could also rest your arms by your sides. Perhaps recite the affirmation: "I trust the strength of my body to hold me today."

# BALASANA

## (RESTORATIVE CHILD'S POSE)

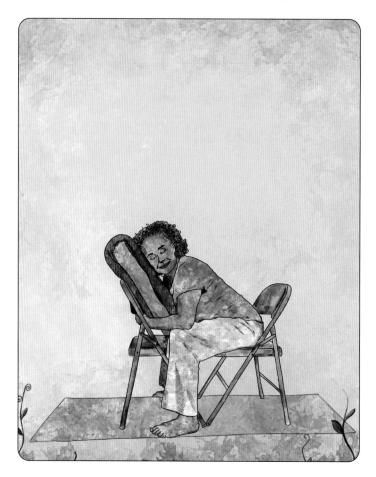

AFFIRMATION: I have always been enough.

INVITATION: If you have a pillow, yoga bolster, or blanket nearby, and you'd like to integrate it into your practice, please feel free to reach for it. If you would like, rest your body over the prop and invite your knees to the outside edges of your mat, if that feels comfortable to you. You can make any adjustments with your arms that feel right, perhaps holding the prop or resting your arms by your sides. You can lay your cheek on the prop and rest here for as long as you need. You can also find a variation with two chairs— sitting on one chair and resting the bolster vertically on the other chair. You could explore hugging the bolster from your seat. Recite the words: "I have always been enough."

# ARM CIRCLES

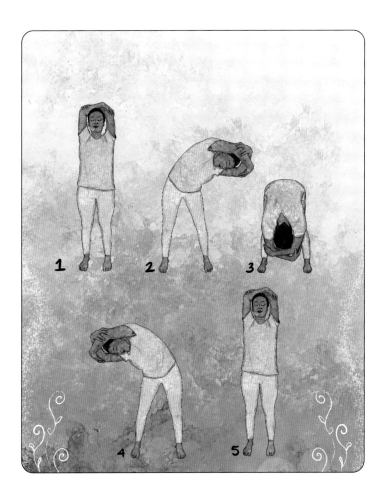

AFFIRMATION: I deserve to live with ease.

INVITATION: Feel free to begin in ragdoll posture. From a standing position, I invite you to release your arms down and interlace your palms, reaching for opposite elbows. If this is hard on your back, please feel free to bend your knees. Perhaps take a moment to honor the symbolism of this posture— releasing anything that does not serve you, your body, your practice, your life. Let it roll off your shoulders and onto the safety and support of the space beneath you. If you would like, find a circular motion with your arms—allowing your inhales to guide you up, and your exhales to circle you down. You deserve to live with ease. Please note this posture is not recommended for people with high blood pressure or eye issues such as glaucoma.

# ADI MUDRA

(FIRST GESTURE)

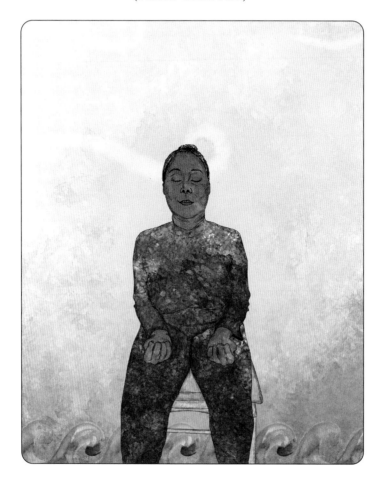

AFFIRMATION: I honor the waves of healing. I can find an anchor amid the storm.

INVITATION: Remember that the choices you make with your body are always celebrated here. Your feelings are valid and important. From a seated posture, I invite you to open your palms and rest your thumbs inside your palms. If it feels okay, wrap your fingers around your thumbs. You are always in choice and in control around how tightly you'd like to grip. Feel free to keep the mudra facing up or down. You might keep your eyes open, close them, or find a soft gaze in front of you. Recite the affirmation to yourself: "I honor the waves of healing. I can find an anchor amid the storm."

# SAVASANA

### (SIDE-LYING OPTION WITH BOLSTER)

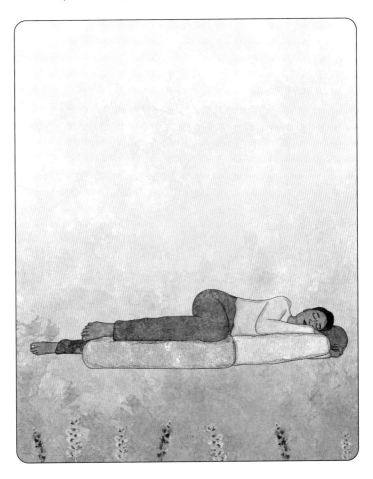

AFFIRMATION: Every time I intentionally choose rest, I know that I am healing. I am held and supported.

INVITATION: Rest is deeply personal. Please know that you can explore any variations of rest that feel accessible to you. If it feels comfortable and available to you, you could rest on your side and perhaps place a bolster or pillow between your knees. You are held and supported.

# HEART-OPENING FLOW

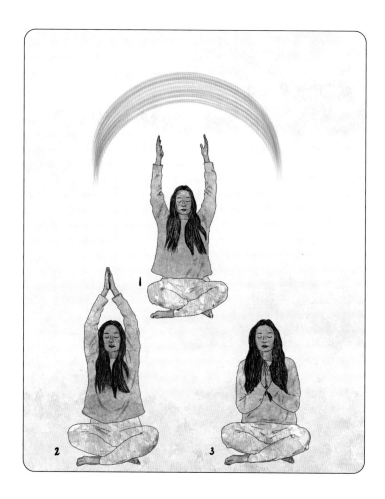

AFFIRMATION: I am creating space for joy.

INVITATION: You could explore this heart-opening posture from
standing or seated. On your inhale breath, I invite you to extend your
arms high to the sky. Notice the strength of your body, the container
it holds for the spectrum of your emotions. Notice your growth as
you extend and find length through your spine and up through your
fingertips. As you feel ready, you might draw your palms together
overhead, if that is available to you. On your exhale, I invite you to
draw your palms through the space of your heart. You could continue
this expression for as long as it feels comfortable. Take note of all of
the space within and around your beautiful body. Maybe even invite
a smile to your face. You are worthy of your own joy.

# ANJALI MUDRA

(SALUTATION SEAL)

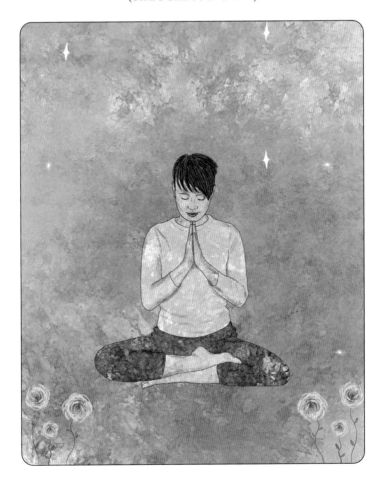

AFFIRMATION: I deserve to take in my own love.

INVITATION: I invite you to find a gesture that symbolizes the love and care you show to yourself. Perhaps it is resting your palms on heart and belly, drawing them together at the space of your heart in Anjali Mudra, or giving yourself a butterfly hug. You could explore a self-compassion or loving-kindness meditation if that feels supportive to you. You are worthy of your own love.

# VIRABHADRASANA II
## (WARRIOR II)

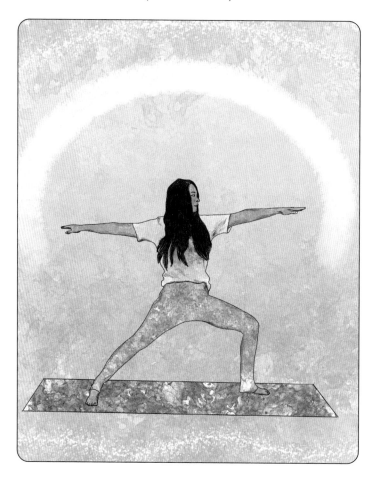

AFFIRMATION: I honor my boundaries.

INVITATION: As your body feels ready, from a standing position, you could explore bending your front knee toward the front of your mat and bringing your back foot parallel to the back of your mat. In your own time and in your own way, you are welcome to extend your arms in each direction—perhaps inviting your gaze forward toward your bent knee. Please feel free to invite any movements that allow this expression to feel more comfortable in your body. I invite you to notice your strength and power. You are worthy of honoring your boundaries.

# VIRABHADRASANA I

(WARRIOR I)

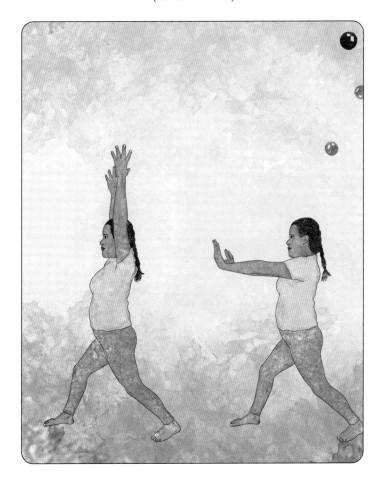

AFFIRMATION: I release what does not serve me.

INVITATION: From a standing posture, feel free to bring your right foot to the front of the mat, slightly bending your right knee if that feels comfortable. I invite you to bring your left foot to the back of the mat, drawing it parallel to your mat. You could explore here with any adjustments to increase your comfort or safety. On your inhale breath, explore an empowering movement of extending your arms to the sky. On your exhale breath, I invite you to push your palms out and away from your body. This is a symbolic gesture of protecting your energy and releasing what does not serve you.

# 5-STEP SELF-HOLDING

(LEVINE, 2008)

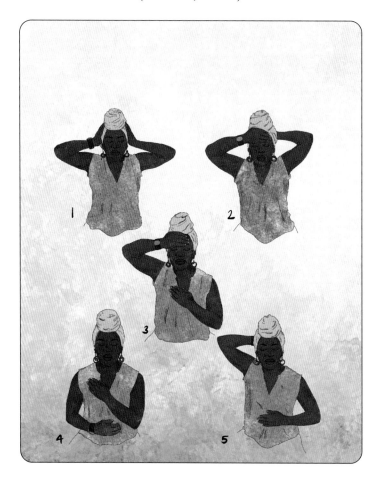

AFFIRMATION: I am resilient. I am home. I am loved. I am in my body.

INVITATION: From a seated position, I invite you to bring both palms to the top of your head. On your inhale breath perhaps bring your right palm over your forehead. On your exhale breath, I invite you to bring your left palm over your heart. On your next inhale breath, perhaps allow your right palm to rest on your belly, and exhale invite your left palm to rest over your right, bringing both palms to your belly. You may want to gently repeat the affirmation to yourself: "I am resilient. I am home. I am loved. I am in my body."

# SETU BANDHA SARVANGASANA

## (SUPPORTED BRIDGE POSE WITH BLOCK)

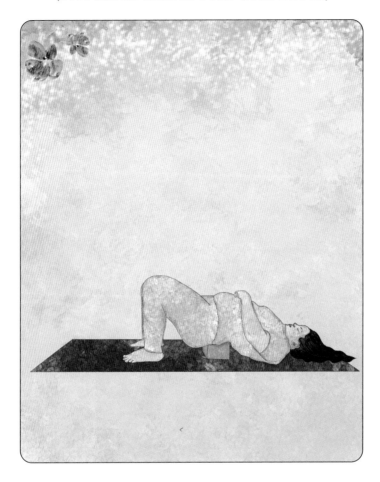

AFFIRMATION: I remember I am worthy of asking for help and receiving support.

INVITATION: When and if it feels safe and accessible in your body, you are welcome to rest on your back, drawing the soles of your feet to the mat and your arms by your side. On your inhale breath, I invite you to lift your hips up and gently slide the block underneath your lower back. On your exhale breath, feel free to melt your sacrum into the block, allowing yourself to feel held and supported. Make any adjustments to increase your comfort. You can remove the block at any time. In this moment remind yourself that you are held, lifted, and supported. You are worthy of asking for help and receiving support.

# SUKHASANA

## (COMFORTABLE POSE)

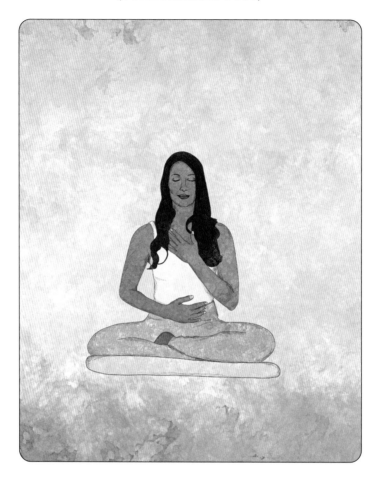

AFFIRMATION: I explore turning the volume of my heart up and the volume of my thoughts down.

INVITATION: If you would like, you can begin in any form of seated that feels supportive in your body. Perhaps on a mat, bolster, or chair. You might explore bringing one hand to your belly and one hand to your heart. I invite you to take a moment to notice the rise and fall of your breath. This is your body and your practice. Take all the time you need. There is no rush. Perhaps recite the affirmation: "I explore turning the volume of my heart up and the volume of my thoughts down."

# ANJALI MUDRA
## (SALUTATION SEAL)

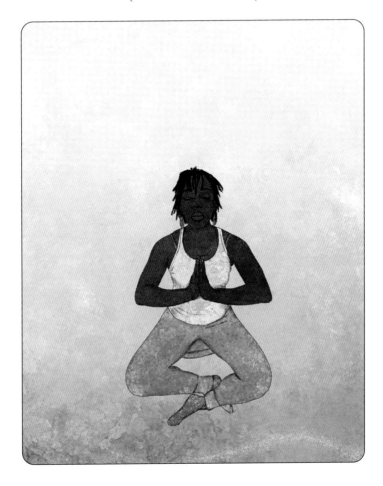

AFFIRMATION: I deserve space to breathe. I am my greatest resource.

INVITATION: I invite you to find a comfortable seated position—perhaps sitting cross-legged, on a cushion, bringing your knees together and sitting on the backs of your heels, or in a chair. Make any adjustments that feel nourishing. Remind yourself that the choices you make with your body are celebrated here. If it feels right, please bring your palms together and rest them in front of your heart. Send yourself gratitude for all the ways you show up for yourself. You are your greatest resource.

# SUKHASANA

(SEATED MEDITATION)

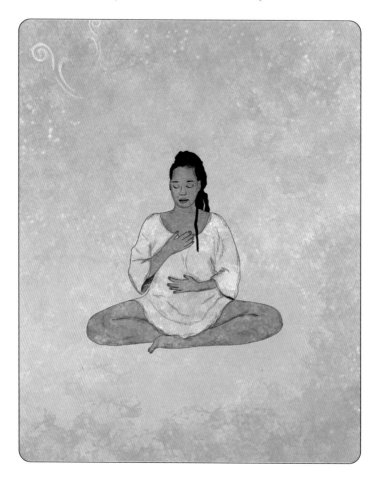

AFFIRMATION: I offer myself patience, kindness, gratitude, and compassion.

INVITATION: If you would like, you can begin in any form of seated that feels right for your body. Perhaps on a mat, bolster, or chair. You might explore bringing one hand to your belly and one hand to your heart. Perhaps take a moment to notice the rise and fall of your breath. I invite you to turn the volume of your heart up and the volume of your thoughts down. This is your body and your practice. Take all the time you need here. There is no rush. Offer yourself patience, kindness, gratitude, and compassion.

# VIRABHADRASANA III

(WARRIOR III)

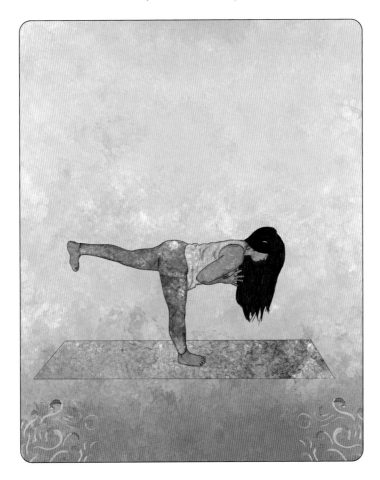

AFFIRMATION: I am not defined by my trauma.

INVITATION: If it feels okay for you, explore balancing on your right foot, and gently draw your fingertips down toward the mat or to a block or book. Extend your left leg back and gently lift it up to the degree that feels comfortable. You could slowly draw your palms together and to the center of your heart. Maybe extend your arms forward to the front of the room like you are making a T shape with your body. Be compassionate with yourself as you explore variations of this posture. That might be keeping your left foot on the mat, or allowing your palms to stay at your heart. Notice the strength within and around you. You are not defined by what has happened to you.

# BHU MUDRA

(EARTH GESTURE)

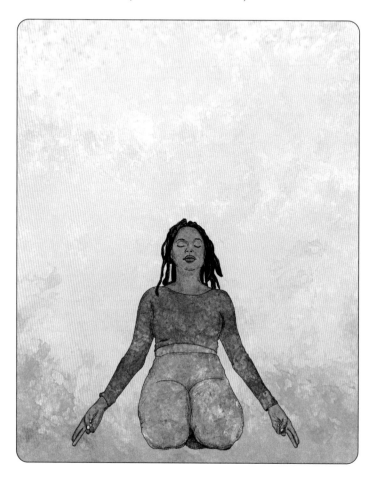

AFFIRMATION: I take mindful moments each day to check in with myself. I offer tenderness and compassion to my nervous system.

INVITATION: From a seated position, I invite you to bring peace fingers to each hand. When you feel ready, perhaps explore grounding your peace fingers into the mat. Invite inhales and exhales at your pace. You could explore drawing your shoulders up and relaxing them down your spine. Practice compassion with your unique experience and recite the affirmation: "I take mindful moments each day to check in with myself. I offer tenderness and compassion to my nervous system."

# BUTTERFLY HUG

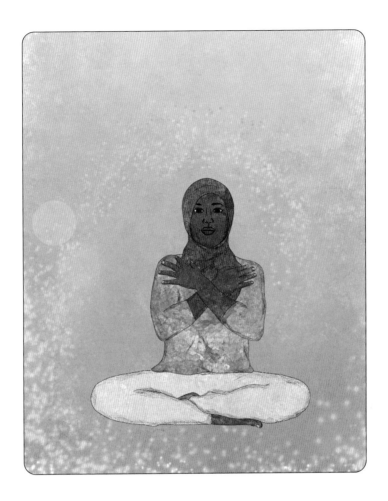

AFFIRMATION: What happened to me was not my fault.

INVITATION: I invite you to find a comfortable seated posture. If it feels right, you could cross your arms across your chest. Perhaps rest the right side of your cheek on your left palm and offer yourself a gentle hug. If it feels safe to continue, please feel free to explore this motion side to side. I invite you to integrate a gentle rocking movement if that feels good for you. I invite you to find a sense of grounding and compassion. What happened to you was not your fault.

# ARDHA SURYA NAMASKAR

## (HALF SUN SALUTATION)

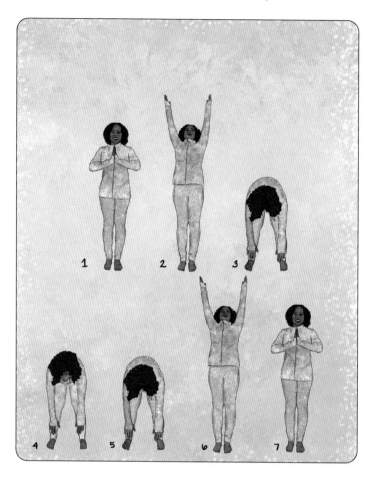

AFFIRMATION: I create routines and rituals that support my mental health.

INVITATION: I invite you to begin in a standing or seated position, whatever might be accessible for you. On your inhale, explore extending your arms high to the sky. Take a moment to notice your feet grounded in your mat or the floor. Know that you are strong and supported—you are never alone in your experience. I invite you to bring your palms together overhead, and on your exhale breath, perhaps make your way to forward fold. On your inhale breath, explore a halfway lift, drawing your palms to your shins, and on your exhale breath, back to forward fold. Continue your sun salutations on your own.

# PADMA MUDRA

## (LOTUS SEAL)

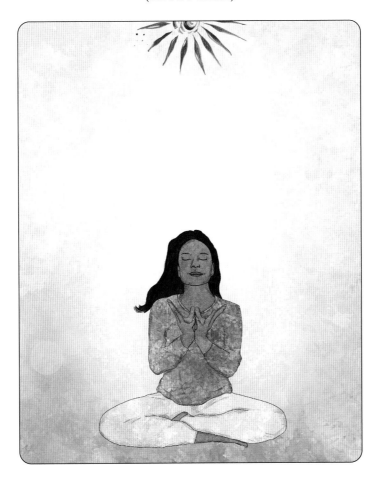

AFFIRMATION: I am innately whole. I draw strength from my resilience.

INVITATION: From a seated posture, I invite you to bring your pinky fingers and thumbs to touch and draw the base of your palms together. From here, perhaps explore unfurling your fingers and extending them upward, much like a lotus would reach for the sky. You are welcome to relax your elbows down and repeat the affirmation: "I am innately whole. I draw strength from my resilience."

# TADASANA

## (SEATED MOUNTAIN)

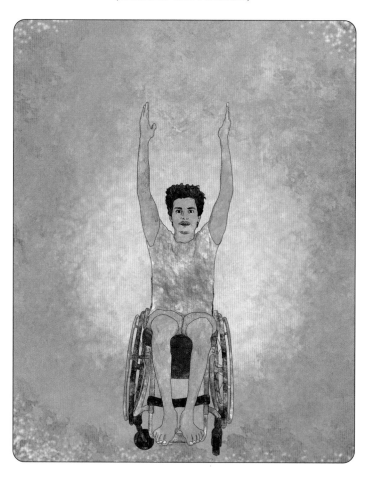

AFFIRMATION: I honor my light.

INVITATION: From a seated posture, I invite you to gently lift your arms to the sky. If it feels comfortable, you might explore facing your palms towards each other and extending your fingertips up. Perhaps take a moment to explore your breath on your terms and relax your shoulders up and back. You might recite the affirmation: "I honor my light."

SUPPORT FOR SURVIVORS ON HOW TO FIND
A TRAUMA-INFORMED YOGA CLASS

I receive a number of inquiries from survivors across the world who are looking for safe spaces to practice. The Breathe Network (http://www.thebreathenetwork.org) is an amazing resource that connects survivors of sexual violence with healing-arts practitioners that offer sliding-scale, trauma-informed, holistic support. Survivors can search by geographic location and/or modality to find practitioners in their area. Additionally, below are questions you might ask of studios, spaces, teachers, or other practitioners to find a place and person that is the right fit for you. You might begin the process of finding a trauma-informed yoga instructor the same way you might approach finding a therapist who is a good fit. Most importantly, trust how interactions with them make you feel when asking questions in person, on the phone, or via email. That may be a powerful indication of your sense of comfort and ease in practicing with them and in their ability to hold space for you.

**Questions to consider:**
- *What is your consent policy around physical assists?*
- *How do you ensure your classes are accessible to those who have experienced trauma?*
- *What does creating safety mean to you?*
- *Do you encourage students to rest and take classes at their own pace?*
- *Do you use supportive and invitational language?*
- *How do you ensure choice is central to the classes you teach?*
- *How do you create an inclusive space in your classes?*
- *Do your teachers receive any form of trauma-informed training during their 200-hour certification?*
- *Do you provide various options for resting in savasana?*
- *How do you cue breath work in your classes?*
- *How do you support students who are triggered?*
- *What does consent look like in your yoga community?*
- *Do you have gender-neutral restrooms?*

Feel free to also spend time journaling your own questions that are unique to you and your lived experience. Don't be afraid to honor your needs, your boundaries, and what is important to you. You are worthy of safety and compassionate support.

## SUPPORT FOR HEALING PROFESSIONALS PREPARING TO TEACH A TRAUMA-INFORMED YOGA CLASS

*Standing or sitting with someone as they realize, remember their own wholeness—that is the work of a healer. . .*
—ADRIENNE MAREE BROWN

If you are taking the steps to begin teaching this modality, I invite you to spend some time reviewing all of the frameworks covered in Chapter 2 and reviewing the guidance on building a curriculum to give you inspiration, ideas, and starting points. You may also want to review the sample script for a trauma-informed yoga class in the appendix.

- Preparing well in advance to teach a trauma-informed yoga class is key. If you have consent or a release of information to review the survivor's intake form, this can give you a sense of what your students are experiencing and how it may inform the way you hold space. For example, your students might be experiencing anxiety, depression, or PTSD, among many other trauma symptoms, and they may also share where they hold trauma in their body.

- You may want to spend some time journaling various themes you hope to cover, but also remain flexible to the needs of your students. They are your greatest teachers. You may have an incredibly thorough and organized plan on the theme of boundaries, but upon entering the space you realize that is not what your students feel ready for. Trust the flow and energy of the space. Honor your students. **Follow their lead.**

- You might carve out time in your schedule to prep for your class while simultaneously turning it into your own self-care time. You could develop your own emotional-safety ritual, create a cozy corner for yourself, play some soft music, drink some tea, and let your inspiration carry you. You might explore free-flow journaling about your class intentions and see what comes up for you. Something that always moves me is thinking about the opportunity I have to center the experiences of those holding the most vulnerable experiences in the room. To do everything I can to ensure they feel seen and reminded that their experience matters.

■ Please see below for some ways to integrate trauma-informed tools into your class preparation. Again, trauma-informed care is not a checklist—it is a lifelong process of honoring the stories of trauma survivors and putting those survivors at the center of their own experience. I hope the invitations below provide a foundation from which to build this work. Please utilize this list in any way that feels supportive to you.

- Does my class sequence include
    - invitational language,
    - variations of postures,
    - accessibility for all bodies,
    - options for resting in savasana,
    - and does it integrate choice and consent throughout?
- Have I been intentional in choosing my quotes, passages, and/or poetry from a diverse range of authors?
- Have I taken time to explain the consent-positive framework around physical assists (permission stones, opting in, no physical assists, consent cards, assist tokens, etc.)?
- Have I dedicated space for students to share community agreements?
- Have I shared where students can access gender-neutral restrooms?
- Have I provided options for students who might experience triggers in class?
- Have I integrated trauma-sensitive breath-work practices?
- Have I asked students about their pronouns?
- Have I invited students to come just as they are?

## Conclusion: Pathways Toward Resilience

*I thought my breathlessness was a sign of my weakness, until a wise friend told me what I wish to tell you: "your breathlessness means you are awake to what's happening right now. The world is in transition.*
—VALARIE KAUR, SEE NO STRANGER

*Say it over and over and over again until you are out of breath. I will not make myself small.*
—UNKNOWN

*I thrive under pressure, yes. But I also thrive under sunshine, under joy, under warm hugs and creativity; morning coffee, a strong community.*

*I can thrive under most things—I'd much rather thrive in love.*
—JOÉL LEON

I can't separate out or categorize the unfathomable things I've been through, nor could I ever capture all of the beauty and overwhelming joy I've been blessed to experience in my life. Each has shaped this journey and made up the fabric of my life. I suppose one of the most profound elements of resilience is the way we learn to embody the intensity of the waves, the nonlinear routes, and honor the strength and light that continues to build within us and trust it as we navigate the storms. Jessica Schaffer defines resilience as "our regulatory capacity to ebb and flow in response to life events" (personal communication, April 2, 2020). I love the flexibility this provides in tending to our healing as an everyday practice. And to be clear, resilience doesn't mean we have to be strong all the time. Resilience offers the gift of vulnerability, the capacity to choose courage in honoring our feelings, and the ability to honor our emotions exactly as they are. More than anything: **You deserve your peace and your spirit is worthy of restoration.** Some of the most profound moments can be found in picking up the broken pieces and putting them back together differently. They represent all the ways you've changed, healed, and continue to heal. They serve as an ongoing reminder of the depth of your heart and your capacity to move through.

I have certainly fallen many times and have had to gather all of the strength around me to get back up again. I vividly remember preparing to give a keynote, Yoga in the Era of #MeToo, at Duke University's Embodied Learning Summit. In the weeks leading up to it I was burning the candle at both ends. Back-to-back trauma trainings. My husband's cancer diagnosis. Relentless work schedule. Navigating crisis. Mothering. Exhaustion. Insomnia. Panic attacks. The ongoing and nonlinear impact to my mental health that is healing from trauma. The voices of "not enough" were loud and visceral.

At the airport, after hearing my name over the loudspeaker because I had left my laptop at security (gives you a sense of how the day was going), I took a deep breath and just let the tears stream down my face. I remember getting on that plane at LAX to North Carolina, gazing out the window and just wondering how it was all going to unfold. I will always be a work in progress but over the years I've learned about the power of trusting our innate gifts and knowledge. The profound wisdom that is woven into the fabric of our stories and our experiences. Learning to trust that wisdom over time has allowed me to take the small, everyday steps to release the perfectionism, the noise, the busy, and the self-induced pressure to overprepare. The ramp-up to big trauma presentations or speaking engagements are often the times I feel the most anxious. The entire process requires me to attend to and nurture my own trauma responses and actually embody the tools and practices that I teach. Each plays a role in the health of my nervous system. There is such power in speaking from our center and grounding ourselves in our own lived experiences. Those truly create a pathway for us to speak from a place of authenticity, courage, emotion, and truth.

I remember walking out to the podium and speaking from that place. And it just flowed right out. No amount of notes, overwhelm, or preparation could replace that. I think our humanness is one of the greatest gifts we can offer one another. So I share the reminder here with you, too. You are worthy of creating space for all of you. You can do hard things with the ease and peace you deserve. Your loving and compassionate presence is more than enough. That weekend my sister also surprised me and flew out to watch my speech and offer her love and support, as she knew what a challenging week I had. Seeing her face in the audience brought me safety and ease.

The entire experience was also a reminder to me that we don't have to push ourselves beyond our limits. Trauma work should be slow and spacious. Yet so many of us work in nonprofit organizations, trauma agencies, universities, or other institutions where we are burned-out, exhausted, carrying caseloads beyond our capacity, and moving at an incredibly unsustainable pace amid everything else we are already holding in our lives. We can't continue like this. We were never designed to function in this capacity. And it has taken years of unpacking those messages to begin to work toward a more grounded way of holding space for survivors. I certainly fall back into patterns that don't serve me, but the gift is in the awareness. That awareness can help inform future choices that are grounded in our own worth and our unique journeys. You might be putting pressure on yourself to heal quickly, but instead, what might it look like to invite in more compassion at a beautiful, slow, steady, and nonlinear pace? I invite you to remind yourself often that you are the expert of you and that there is absolutely no rush to your healing.

The thing that always moves me about healing is how small and subtle, yet powerful, the shifts are over time. The ways we start to step into our own power, truth, value, and worth and make intentional choices around our own care. Sometimes the impact of healing feels tangible and other times it's an overarching lightness in the way we move through the world.

Healing is not linear, and I also celebrate the moments when I choose to honor my strength, my journey, and my desire not to shrink. Healing has given me the gift of awareness and has helped me create a pathway that no longer requires me to diminish my spirit or accept that living in survival mode is the only answer.

I'm on a journey to finding more rest in my life, more space, more ease, more breath, more gentleness.

To anyone who needs the reminder: you deserve to honor the fullness of your truth, your journey, your value, your care, and your needs. Your well-being matters.

You have so much to offer this world. And you don't have to wait for anyone to tell you that. **You are capable and you are ready.** I hope this book has provided you with a landscape for you to begin to paint your own canvas of healing and/or continue to meaningfully impact the lives of the survivors you have the honor of holding space for. I hope it continues to serve as a soft place to land. A supportive resource and also an affirming reminder that you are worthy of your dreams and your healing.

May this be your reminder to trust the power of your innate resilience. **You have always been enough, exactly as you are.**

# Sample Trauma-Informed Yoga Class Script

**Theme: Trust in your gifts and your healing.**

Today I invite you to find grounding in your worthiness. Feel free to begin in any shape that supports the safety of your body. Take up all of the space you deserve and remind yourself that you are worthy of this time. Know that the choices you make with your own body are celebrated in this space. You have already done the hardest work of arriving. Send yourself a moment of gratitude for all of the ways you show up for you.

KNOW THAT EVERYTHING is optional and you can opt out at any time. This is your body and always your practice. This is your window of time to honor you and your needs.

FEEL FREE TO get started in any form of rest that feels comfortable in your body. Rest is deeply personal, so feel free to find a shape that supports your safety. Know that you can keep your eyes open, find a soft focus on anything in front of you, or close the eyes—whatever feels most safe for you.

IF IT FEELS comfortable to you, you could explore resting on your back with a pillow or bolster underneath your knees, allowing your arms to fall by your sides. Perhaps allow a gentle relaxation through your shoulders—inviting them to nestle into the safety and support of your yoga mat. If you prefer, you can explore lying on your favorite side—feel free to use any props to support you in finding a shape within your body that feels authentic for you. If you'd like you can draw the soles of your feet to the mat, lie on your belly, make your way to Child's Pose, or find any other shape that is calling you. If sitting up feels better, please respect and honor wherever your body is today.

AND MOST IMPORTANTLY, know that there is nothing left to do. You made it to your mat and sometimes that is the hardest part. Honor your body. Honor your breath. I invite you to drop into this moment. Letting go of your day, letting go of any distractions, letting go of whatever it took for you to get here today. If you wanted to find one posture that really resonates with you and stay there for the entire class, that would be perfect and supported. This is your body and always your practice. Allow this to be a gentle space for you, your body, your needs, and your breath. Perhaps invite the embodied feeling of being held or supported. You are never alone in your experience.

THIS EXPERIENCE IS about making conscious choices for your body. Listening to the needs of your body and responding in ways that feel kind and compassionate to you. I invite you to breathe in and out at your pace.

I INVITE YOU to spend a few moments quieting the mind and gently finding connection to your breath. You could explore turning the volume of your heart up and the volume of your thoughts down. Feel free to inhale and exhale in a way that feels natural. No need to constrict your breathing in any way.

PERHAPS BRING AWARENESS to any sensations flowing through your body. Maybe notice the level of physical or emotional energy you are bringing to your mat today. There is no need to fix or change anything, just notice. Maybe listen to the sound of your own breath and breathe in a way that feels accessible to you.

I INVITE YOU to set an intention for your practice. What do you need more of in this moment? Perhaps reciting a mantra or affirmation is something that resonates with you today. You can repeat this as many times as you would like. If at any time being with the internal sensations in your body feels like too much, you are always welcome to focus on something external in the space. This could be a sound, color, scent—anything that feels grounding or supports you in reorienting back to the safety of your space.

WHAT DOES IT look like here in our practice to hold the many paradoxes of healing? To honor the grief, but also make space for abundant joy. What does it feel like to ride the waves of healing as they come? What if we could be compassionate with ourselves when we tap into the deep knowing that there may be no finish line to this thing called healing. Can we hold on fiercely to our worthiness amid the many storms we will inevitably encounter in this life? Can we let ourselves be present with moments of relief and joy? And can we consciously practice self-love and know that, in the beautiful words of Alex Elle:

"WE CAN BE whole and still be discovering pieces of ourselves. Resilient and still sensitive. Learning and still making mistakes along the way. Growing and still working through grief. Healing and still need support."

(Alex Elle, @alexelle, Instagram, August 28, 2018)

When your body feels ready, there is absolutely no rush—I invite you to gently invite the movement and awareness back into your body. Perhaps begin with wiggling out your toes, circling out your ankles, bringing movement into your fingers, circling out your wrists. Maybe explore interlacing your arms overhead, finding a wall-to-wall stretch.

**Continue with trauma-informed cues**

    Supine twist

    Seated meditation and hip circles

    Neck rolls

    Shoulder rolls

    5-Step Self-Holding (Levine, 2008)

    Seated meditation with Adi Mudra

    Gateway Pose

    Downward-Facing Dog or straight to standing

    Ragdoll

    Arm circles

## SAMASTITIHI

I invite you to draw the palms together at heart center if that feels comfortable for you. Maybe rub your palms together to allow the heat to radiate. If it feels okay, place those palms over your heart.

**Read quote**

*Most of my life has been spent trying to shrink myself. Trying to become smaller. Quieter. Less sensitive. Less opinionated. Less needy. Less me. Because I didn't want to be a burden. I didn't want to be too much or push people away. I wanted people to like me. I wanted to be cared for and valued. I wanted to be wanted. So for years, I sacrificed myself for the sake of making other people happy. And for years, I suffered. But I'm tired of suffering, and I'm done shrinking. It's not my job*

*to change who I am in order to become someone else's idea*
*of a worthwhile human being. I am worthwhile. Not because*
*other people think I am, but because I exist, and therefore I*
*matter. My thoughts matter. My feelings matter. My voice mat-*
*ters. And with or without anyone's permission or approval, I will*
*continue to be who I am and speak my truth. Even if it makes*
*people angry. Even if it makes them uncomfortable. Even if they*
*choose to leave. I refuse to shrink. I choose to take up space. I*
*choose to honor my feelings. I choose to give myself permis-*
*sion to get my needs met. I choose to make* **self-care** *a priority.*
*I choose me.*

—DANIELL KOEPKE,
 ORIGINALLY PUBLISHED IN
 *DARING TO TAKE UP SPACE* (2020)

I invite you to breathe all of that in and exhale out. Let's explore taking three breaths here to unite our community, to unite our practice—to unite our collective intentions in the room.

## SUN SALUTATION A

(slow pace, continue trauma-informed cues) Inhale—Mountain Pose—extend your energy and intention high to the sky—offer it up; exhale—backbend—allow your heart to shine bright; inhale—Mountain Pose; exhale—forward fold; inhale—halfway lift; exhale—forward fold (repeat as many times as you'd like, inviting students to explore their own expression and variations of the movements)

## Read quote

*And through it all, what a gift you give to this world by choosing*
*to remain open.*
—DANIELLE DOBY

## CHILD'S POSE

You are welcome to massage your forehead into the mat or explore stretching your arms left and right—creating more space in your side body. Take as much time as you need to rest here. When you feel ready, you are welcome to make your way to downward-facing dog if that feels comfortable for you.

## CHAIR POSE

sweep arms left and side—to release fear, self-doubt, shame, etc.


Invitation to move through Sun Salutation A to downward facing dog

> Right leg high
> Low lunge to side twist
> Back to low lunge
> Warrior I—with palms push out energy that does not serve you
> Warrior II
> Reverse Warrior
> Repeat 2x
> Child's Pose


### Read quote

*You can be healed and still healing. You can be open and still hurting. You can be brave and still frightened.*

—REBECCA RAY,
    EXCERPT FROM *THE UNIVERSE LISTENS TO BRAVE*.
    COPYRIGHT REBECCA RAY, 2019. REPRINTED WITH PERMISSION
    FORM PUBLISHER.


> Runner's Lunge
> Pigeon Pose
> Paschimottanasana—forward fold
> Bhu Mudra
> Supported Bridge
> Savasana

As it feels right, start to draw the awareness back in. Maybe wiggling out your fingers and circling out your wrists, perhaps wiggling out your toes and circling out the ankles. Gently bring the sensations and awareness back into your body. At your own pace, feel free to meet me in a seated position.

I invite you to bring the heels of your palms together, drawing your pinkies and thumbs together, allowing the fingers to blossom open like a lotus. The lotus flower blooms on the surface of the water, with its roots deep below the mud—making it a symbol for light emerging from darkness. You represent this beautiful light. If you'd like, bring your palms to your heart. Hands at your heart, may we live our lives compassionately; hands at your mouth, may we speak words of truth and of kindness; and hands at your third-eye center, may the light in me, honor the light in you. Bowing forward to seal your practice, to seal the magic we created in the room. Namaste.

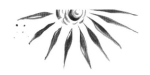

# TEACHING PHILOSOPHY

Teaching trauma-informed yoga, creating restorative and safe spaces, inviting opportunities for more softness and rest are the work of my heart. My promise to you as a teacher:

.................

I will hold the container with the utmost compassion and honor all of the ways in which trauma impacts the mind, body, and spirit.

.................

I honor the pace of each of our journeys and hold the deep knowing that our experiences are different, messy, nuanced, and beautiful. There is no one-size-fits-all approach. I welcome you exactly as you are.

.................

I honor the pace in which you are able to engage with the material and with your body. You are in control of what feels best for you. I'm here to support you every step of the way.

.................

I honor the concept of working toward an embodied sense of safety and boundaries. We will work together to create a space where you can safely attend to the physiological messages of your body and honor self- and community care.

..................

I am acutely aware that many of us come to this work with experiences of trauma. This requires that we be extra gentle with ourselves. That we don't have to have it all figured out. That we can be honest when listening is hard. Taking what you need moment to moment will always be celebrated.

..................

There are no hierarchies in this journey. We are co-creating and learning from each other. Your lived experience is your greatest teacher.

..................

I believe in the palpable stories our bodies hold and in our ability to gently uncover, tend to, and nurture them. I promise to provide multiple choices and support you in feeling seen and experiencing ease.

# ACKNOWLEDGMENTS

*Oh, the comfort, the inexpressible comfort of feeling safe with a person; having neither to weigh thoughts nor measure words, but to pour them all out, just as they are, chaff and grain together, knowing that a faithful hand will take and sift them, keep what is worth keeping, and then, with a breath of kindness, blow the rest away.*
—GEORGE ELIOT

### WE WERE NEVER MEANT TO DO THIS ALONE

I am forever grateful to the village that kept me lifted and held throughout this entire writing and (inevitable healing process).

### TO MY DARLING HUSBAND, GARRETT YAMASAKI

You are an unbelievable rock. You are the calm to my anxiety and the anchor in every storm. Sometimes I wonder what I did to deserve a love like yours. You have loved me through the depths of my healing and our vows from that little Japanese garden wedding still ring true each and every day. You have held me and seen me through two pregnancies and two deliveries. You have taught me the meaning and the nuances of the word "unconditional." I am forever grateful for the most perfect cup of coffee (and forehead kisses) that you make each morning and the many cups you made to help me get through my writing slumps! You nourish me in ways I alone could never have the capacity for. Thank you for reminding me every single day that I am enough and that my trauma does not define me. Thank you for championing me and celebrating every accomplishment. Thank you for teaching me to cherish joy in the little things and practice gratitude. You are one of a kind and I love your heart. You are an incredible partner, father, son, brother, friend, coach, photographer—and so much more. I know this is just the beginning of the many adventures that life has in store for us. I adore your heart and love you deeply.

### TO MY BEAUTIFUL SON, HUDSON

You are pure light and joy. You have made all of my dreams come true and your smile has been a balm to so many wounds. Thank you for being the sweetest healer and giving me strength to finish this book when you were just 2 years old. One day you will look back and read this and realize all the ways you have wrapped my heart. You are mine, we are one. I can't wait to see all you will do in this world just for being you, exactly as you are. Mama loves you so much.

### TO MY PARENTS, RIZWANA AND AKBAR

I feel emotional as I write this but I am infinitely grateful for the power of your love. For supporting my passions every step of the way. You've been the most beautiful role models and examples of what is possible when you believe in yourself. Your hard work, your story, and your selflessness have inspired me my whole life. Thank you for your compassion and for helping me amid so many moments of overwhelm. Thank you for creating the life and opportunities you have for Almina and me. We owe it all to you. Thank you for believing in me. Thank you for getting pens and tote bags made with my logo. Your love has made me whole.

### TO MY SISTER, ALMINA

There are no words to describe our bond and all the ways your companionship has brought me joy. Thank you for all the ways you have helped me build my strength and confidence. Thank you for traveling across the country multiple times to be with me when I needed you most. Thank you for your daily texts of support. Thank you for your gentle guidance. Thank you for protecting me on the playground when we were little girls and for fiercely protecting me every day since. You are an incredible inspiration, an amazing mom, sister, daughter, wife, among so many identities you hold. Thank you for reminding me to love myself.

### TO MY MOTHER- AND FATHER-IN-LAW, BARBARA AND JAMES

I am so blessed to be a part of this family. Your generosity, loyalty, love, and unconditional support are present in more ways than I could ever capture. You are truly the kindest, most giving humans and your support of this book and all of my work has meant so much to my heart. Thank you for taking care and loving on Hudson during my stressful moments of deadlines and overwhelm! There is no one in the world like you both.

### TO MY SISTER-IN-LAW, SHANNON

May you always believe in yourself and all that you are capable of. Your love and loyalty are just a few of the many qualities that make you the incredible human you are. Your mothering inspires me daily. I am in awe of all you are and all you do.

### TO MY BEST FRIENDS JENNY, JULES, MEGAN, AND SAM

I love and adore you all. Your grace, unbelievable support, daily check-ins, and wisdom have carried me in my darkest times. Our seventeen years of friendship have filled my heart with hope and inspiration. I am forever grateful to have you by my side.

### TO MY POWERFUL SOUL SISTERS, HEALERS, COLLEAGUES, AND FRIENDS

Allyson P., Azita, Caitlin, Cora, Debbie, Eve, Jess H., Jessica H., Jody, Karla, Kelsey, La Shonda, Lilian, Marian, Molly B., Molly N., Nadeeka, Nicole Q., Nikita, Nityda, Shena, Smita, and Whitney: I can't believe how lucky I am to be surrounded by such powerful and inspiring women, who truly show me each and every day that anything is possible. The light that each of you shines is remarkable. I am grateful to learn from you and to have your powerful presence in my life. My gratitude for you is endless. You have been the most beautiful support system amid the many ebbs and flows of my life. And your sisterhood has carried me through each storm. I love you so much.

## TO MY DEAR EVE

I don't know how I could possibly capture in words what you mean to me. "I love you" doesn't even capture it. You are radiant, resilient, nurturing, brilliant, and brave. You are a survivor in all the ways the word embodies. You are an incredible mother, partner, friend, sister, daughter, ally, and artist. Our bond and connection knows no bounds. Thank you for creating the most breathtaking images for this book and the affirmation deck. This collaboration has brought me profound joy. May you never forget the power of your light and your gifts. You inspire me every single day.

## TO MY DEAR SHENA

My beautiful Shena, boo. Wow. What a journey we have traveled together. I feel emotional when I think of you because you remind me of pure goodness, beauty, and light. Your heart is beautiful. May you always remember your worth, your profound gifts, and all you have to offer. "I Am Light" by India Arie will always remind me of you and it brings the biggest smile to my face. I feel so blessed to travel the journey of healing with you, to do this work alongside each other, to support each other with our whole hearts. Thank you for writing an inspiring foreword for this book. There is not a day I take our friendship for granted. I love you. I am so happy you exist.

## TO MY AMAZING ASSISTANTS, HALEY AND TOSHA

There are no words to possibly capture the ease and comfort you have brought to my life. I certainly would not be functioning without you! I am so blessed for your grace and compassion in my life. Thank you for managing all that you do and for making it possible for me to manage all of the pieces of this book. I am so grateful for you.

**TO MY COLLEAGUE AND FRIEND, DAVID TRELEAVEN**

Without your support and direction, I would not be here. Thank you for believing in me before I believed in myself. Thank you for making this dream come true. Thank you for responding to my novel text messages with clarity, guidance, love, and support. And thank you for writing one of the beautiful forewords of this book. Keep sharing your gifts and wisdom with the world. We need your light.

**TO THE TEAM AT NORTON**

Thank you, Deborah, for your enthusiastic support of this book from the very beginning, for your unbridled encouragement, and for keeping me motivated and supported along the way. Thank you to the entire team at Norton for your compassionate support and guidance and for making this dream a reality. I am eternally grateful.

**TO EVERYONE WHO PARTICIPATED IN THE ILLUSTRATIONS FOR THE BOOK**

Thank you for sharing your spirit with us and for helping bring this healing resource to life.

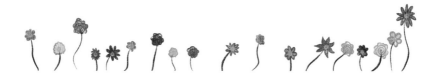

# RESOURCES

## Recommended Reading

*Accessible Yoga*, Jivana Heyman

*Accessing the Healing Power of the Vagus Nerve*, Stanley Rosenberg

*Attachment-Based Yoga and Meditation for Trauma Recovery*, Deirdre Fay

*Emotional Yoga*, Bija Bennett

*Hood Feminism: Notes From the Women That a Movement Forgot*, Mikki Kendall

*How to Be an Antiracist*, Ibram X. Kendi

*How to Breathe*, Ashley Neese

*Joyous Resilience*, Anjuli Sherin

*Meditations for Healing Trauma*, Louanne Davis

*Mindfulness-Oriented Interventions for Trauma: Integrating Contemplative Practices*, Victoria M. Follette, John Briere, Deborah Rozelle, James W. Hopper, and David I. Rome (editors)

*Mindfulness Skills for Trauma and PTSD: Practices for Recovery and Resilience*, Rachel Goldsmith Turow

*Mindfulness Therapy Workbook for Clinicians and Clients*, C. Alexander Simpkins and Annellen M. Simpkins

*Mindful of Race: Transforming Racism From the Inside Out*, Ruth King

*My Grandmother's Hands*, Resmaa Menakem

*Occupy This Body: A Buddhist Memoir*, Sharon Suh

*Overcoming Trauma Through Yoga: Reclaiming Your Body*, David Emerson

*Radiant Rest*, Tracee Stanley

*Radical Dharma: Talking Race, Love, and Liberation*, Rev. angel Kyodo williams, Lama Rod Owens, and Jasmine Syedullah

*Restorative Yoga for Ethnic and Race-Based Stress and Trauma*, Dr. Gail Parker

*Set Boundaries, Find Peace,* Nedra Glover Tawwab

*Skill in Action*, Michelle Cassandra Johnson

*Survivors on the Yoga Mat*, Becky Thompson

*The Art of Healing From Sexual Trauma*, Naomi Ardea

*The Body Keeps the Score: Brain, Mind, and Body in the Healing of Trauma*, Bessel van der Kolk

*The Inner Work of Racial Justice*, Rhonda V. Magee

*The iRest Program for Healing PTSD: A Proven Effective Approach to Using Yoga Nidra Meditation and Deep Relaxation Techniques to Overcome Trauma*, Richard C. Miller

*The Mindful Self-Compassion Workbook*, Kristin Neff and Christopher Germer
*The Power of Breathwork*, Jennifer Patterson
*Trauma and the Body*, Pat Ogden, Kekuni Minton, and Clare Pain
*Trauma-Sensitive Mindfulness*, David Treleaven
*Trauma-Sensitive Yoga in Therapy: Bringing the Body Into Treatment*, David Emerson
*Trauma to Dharma*, Dr. Azita Nahai
*Waking the Tiger: Healing Trauma*, Peter Levine
*Yoga for Emotional Balance*, Bo Forbes
*Yoga for Grief and Loss: Poses, Meditation, Devotion, Self-Reflection, Selfless Acts, Ritual*, Karla Helbert
*Yoga for Trauma Recovery*, Lisa Danylchuk
*Yoga Skills for Therapists*, Amy Weintraub

## Social Justice and Trauma-Informed Yoga Educators, Therapists, and Healers

### EDUCATORS, YOGA INSTRUCTORS, AND HEALERS
Amy Weintraub, https://yogafordepression.com/
Amy Wheeler, https://amywheeler.com/
Aurea Victoria, https://aureavictoria.com/
Bo Forbes, https://boforbes.com/
Chelsea Jackson Roberts, http://www.chelsealovesyoga.com/
De Jur Jones, https://www.idreaminyoga.com/
Devin Grindrod, http://spirituallybalanced.com/
Dianne Bondy, https://diannebondyyoga.com/
Dr. Gail Parker, https://www.drgailparker.com/
Erica Rey, https://www.ericarey.com
Eve Andry, https://www.eveandry.com/
Hala Khouri, https://halakhouri.com/
Jacoby Ballard, https://jacobyballard.net/about/
Jamie Hanson, https://jamiehansonyoga.com/
Jasmine Allen, https://withjasmineallen.com/
Jill Weiss, https://www.yogaforhealingtrauma.com
Katrina Long, https://manifestingmewellness.com
Kimberly Ann Johnson, https://www.magamama.com/
Lisa Danylchuk, https://lisadanylchuk.com/
Michelle Cassandra Johnson, https://www.michellecjohnson.com/
Molly Boeder Harris, http://www.mollyboederharris.com/
Nicole Steward, https://www.radical-tendencies.com/
Nityda Gessel, https://traumaconsciousyoga.com/meet-nityda/
Octavia Raheem, https://octaviaraheem.com/
Rachel Allen, http://www.yogasong.net
Ryann Summers, https://www.ryannsummersyoga.com/
Sanaz Yaghmai, https://www.alchemyoftrauma.com/

Sarah Savino (Instagram), https://www.instagram.com/the_fit_philanthropist/
Sarit Z. Rogers, https://saritzrogers.com/
Shena Young, http://www.embodiedtruthhealing.com/
Susanna Barkataki, https://www.susannabarkataki.com/
Tarana Burke, https://metoomvmt.org/
Tara Tonini, https://www.taratonini.com/

## ORGANIZATIONS

Amita Swadhin, Mirror Memoirs, http://mirrormemoirs.com
Anna Smith, Hope Bound Collective, https://www.hopeboundcollective.com
Black Emotional and Mental Health Collective, https://www.beam.community
Coaching for Healing, Justice, and Liberation, https://www.healingjusticeliberation.org
Echo, https://www.echotraining.org
Elevate Uplift, Circle of Wisdom, https://www.elevateuplift.org/circleofwisdom
Empowered Spaces, https://empoweredspaces.net
Exhale to Inhale, https://www.exhaletoinhale.org
Firecracker Foundation, https://thefirecrackerfoundation.org
Integrate Network, http://www.letsintegrate.org
iRest, https://www.irest.org
Jivana Heyman, Accessible Yoga, https://accessibleyoga.org
Just Detention International, https://www.justdetention.org
Molly Boeder Harris, The Breathe Network, http://www.thebreathenetwork.org
Monsoon Asians & Pacific Islanders in Solidarity https://monsooniowa.org
National Organization of Asians and Pacific Islanders Ending Sexual Violence https://napiesv.org
National Queer and Trans Therapists of Color Network, https://www.nqttcn.com
Nikki Myers, Yoga of 12-Step Recovery, https://y12sr.com
Nkem Ndefo, Lumos Transforms, https://lumostransforms.com
Uprising Yoga, https://www.uprisingyoga.org
Yoga for Eating Disorders, https://www.yoga4eatingdisorders.com

## SUPPORTIVE SOCIAL MEDIA ACCOUNTS (INSTAGRAM)

@alex_elle
@asianwomencollegesurvivors
@chanel_miller
@chaninicholas
@cleowade
@decolonizingtherapy
@dr.yaghmai
@dr.thema
@embodiedtruthhealing
@embody.create.heal
@freefromdotorg
@grounded_and_guided_yoga
@healingfromptsd
@heathertuba

@inclusivetherapists
@integrate_network
@kindredmedicine
@_lisaolivera
@melaninandmentalhealth
@metoomvmt
@minaa_b
@mirror.memoirs
@morganharpernichols
@movementforhealing
@nedratawwab
@nsvrc
@recipesforselflove
@rootsofsouthla
@somewhere_under_the_rainbow
@susannabarkataki
@taranajaneen
@the_traumatherapist
@thebreathenetwork
@theempoweredtherapist
@thefirecrackerfoundation
@thenapministry
@transcending_trauma_with_yoga
@trauma_conscious_yoga_method
@trauma.informed.yoga
@trauma.sensitive.mindfulness
@traumaandco
@traumaawarecare
@traumainformedla
@valariekaur

## TRAUMA-INFORMED AND SOMATIC THERAPISTS
Anjuli Sherin, https://www.anjulisherinmft.com
Dr. Azita Nahai, https://azitanahai.com/about/
Dr. Deborah Schleicher, https://www.westlosangelespsychologist.com/
Dr. Mandy Mount, https://www.psychologytoday.com/us/therapists/mandy-mount
    -irvine-ca/372368
Dr. Thema, https://www.drthema.com/
Dr. Whitney Dicterow, https://www.drwhitneydicterow.com/
Jody Barnes, https://www.jodybarnes.com/
Linda Crossley, https://sanctuary4compassion.com/
Maggie MacLeod, https://www.dandelionintegrativetherapy.com/

## YOGA AND TRAUMA EVIDENCE-BASED RESEARCH ARTICLES

Desikachar, K., Bragdon, L., & Bossart, C. (2005). The yoga of healing: Exploring yoga's holistic model for health and well-being. *International Journal of Yoga Therapy*, *15*, 17–39.

Dick, A. M., Niles, B. L., Street, A. E., DiMartino, D. M., & Mitchell, K. S. (2014). Examining mechanisms of change in a yoga intervention for women: The influence of mindfulness, psychological flexibility, and emotion regulation on PTSD symptoms. *Journal of Clinical Psychology*, *70*(12), 1170–1182.

Draucker, C. B., Martsolf, D. S., Ross, R., Cook, C. B., Stidham, A. W., & Mweemba, P. (2009). The essence of healing from sexual violence: A qualitative metasynthesis. *Research in Nursing & Health*, *32*(4), 366–378.

Elliott, D. E., Bjelajac, P., Fallot, R. D., Markoff, L. S., & Reed, B. G. (2005). Trauma-informed or trauma-denied: Principles and implementation of trauma-informed services for women. *Journal of Community Psychology*, *33*(4), 461–477.

Emerson, D., Sharma, R., Chaudhry, S., & Turner, J. (2009). Trauma-sensitive yoga: Principles, practice, and research. *International Journal of Yoga Therapy*, *19*, 123–128.

Macy, R. J., Jones, E., Graham, L. M., & Roach, L. (2018). Yoga for trauma and related mental health problems: A meta-review with clinical and service recommendations. *Trauma, Violence, & Abuse*, *19*(1), 35–57.

Mitchell, K. S., Dick, A. M., DiMartino, D. M., Smith, B. N., Biles, B., Koenen, K. C., & Street, A. (2014). A pilot study of a randomized controlled trial of yoga as an intervention for PTSD symptoms in women. *Journal of Traumatic Stress*, *27*, 121–128.

Reeves, E. (2015). A synthesis of the literature on trauma-informed care. *Issues in Mental Health Nursing*, *36*(9), 698–709.

Rhodes, A., Spinazzola, J., & van der Kolk, B. (2016). Yoga for adult women with chronic PTSD: A long-term follow-up study. *The Journal of Alternative and Complementary Medicine*, *22*(3).

Schweitzer, M., Gilpin, L., & Frampton, S. (2004). Healing spaces: Elements of environmental design that make an impact on health. *The Journal of Alternative and Complementary Medicine*, *10*(1), 71–83.

Telles, S. (2012). Managing mental health disorders resulting from trauma through yoga: A review. *Depression Research and Treatment*, *2012*, 1–9.

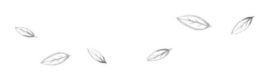

# REFERENCES

Altman, J. (2007). Releasing the Tangles of Trauma through Body-energy Healing. *Self & Society, 34*(4), 5–12. https://doi.org/10.1080/03060497.2007.11083926

Black, M. C., Basile, K. C., Breiding, M. J., Smith, S. G., Walters, M. L., Merrick, M. T., Chen, J., & Stevens, M. R. (2011). The National Intimate Partner and Sexual Violence Survey (NISVS): 2010 Summary Report. Atlanta, GA: National Center for Injury Prevention and Control, Centers for Disease Control and Prevention.

Boeder Harris, M. (2013). *Reintegrating the body, mind & spirit after sexual violence.* Elephant. https://www.elephantjournal.com/2013/08/reintegrating-the-body-mind-spirit-after-sexual-violence-molly-boeder-harris/

Boeder Harris, M. (2015, July 11). Trauma Informed Yoga – Savasana [Video]. YouTube. https://youtu.be/fPthXHmRSrs

Boeder Harris, M. (2015, July 12). http://www.thebreathenetwork.org/shining-a-trauma-informed-lens-on-yoga-savasana

Brown, A. M. (2017). *Emergent Strategy: Shaping Change, Changing Worlds* (Reprint ed.). AK Press.

Building Cultures of Care: A Guide for Sexual Assault Services Programs. (2017). Retrieved 2020, from Nsvrc.org website: https://www.nsvrc.org/sites/default/files/2017-10/publications_nsvrc_building-cultures-of-care.pdf

Butler, L. D., Critelli, F. M., & Rinfrette, E. S. (2011). Trauma-informed care and mental health. *Directions in Psychiatry, 31*(3), 177–192.

Campbell, R. (2014). *The world's messiest desk* [video]. YouTube. https://www.youtube.com/watch?v=vdx2E5wArt8

Campbell, R., Sefl, T., & Athens, C. E. (2003). The physical health consequences of rape: Assessing survivors' somatic symptoms in a racially diverse population. *Women's Studies Quarterly, 31* (1/2), 99–104.

Carter, R. T., Ph.D. (2015, May 28). *Race & Trauma: Race-Based Traumatic Stress and Psychological Injury* [Slides]. The Community Technical Assistance Center of New York. https://www.ctacny.org/sites/default/files/trainings-pdf/race_%26_trauma_5.28.15.final_.pdf

Clark, C., Lewis-Dmello, A., Anders, D., Parsons, A., Nguyen-Feng, V., Henn, L., & Emerson, D. (2014). Trauma-sensitive yoga as an adjunct mental health treatment in group therapy for survivors of domestic violence: A feasibility study. HHS Public Access. https://www.ncbi.nlm.nih.gov/pmc/articles/PMC4215954/

Cleary, M., & Hungerford, C. (2015). Trauma-informed Care and the Research Literature: How Can the Mental Health Nurse Take the Lead to Support Women Who Have Survived Sexual Assault? *Issues in Mental Health Nursing, 36*(5), 370–378. https://doi.org/10.3109/01612840.2015.1009661

Criswell, E., Wheeler, A., & Partlow Lauttamus, M. (2014). Yoga Therapy Research, Individualized Yoga Therapy and Call It Yoga Therapy. *International Journal of Yoga Therapy, 24*(1), 23–29. https://doi.org/10.17761/ijyt.24.1.a472jr148535634j

Danylchuk, L. (2019). *Yoga for trauma recovery: Theory, philosophy, and practice.* Routledge.

Davidson, M. M. (2019). *Exploring the Efficacy of Trauma-Informed Yoga for Survivors of Sexual Assault on College Campuses.* Unpublished manuscript.

Davis, L. (1990). *The Courage to Heal Workbook: A Guide for Women and Men Survivors of Child Sexual Abuse* (1st ed.). Harper Perennial.

Dick, A. M., Niles, B. L., Street, A. E., DiMartino, D. M., & Mitchell, K. S. (2014). Examining mechanisms of change in a yoga intervention for women: The influence of mindfulness, psychological flexibility, and emotion regulation on PTSD symptoms. *Journal of Clinical Psychology, 70*(12), 1170–1182.

Elliott, D. E., Bjelajac, P., Fallot, R. D., Markoff, L. S., & Reed, B. G. (2005). Trauma-informed or trauma-denied: Principles and implementation of trauma-informed services for women. *Journal of Community Psychology, 33*(4), 461–477. https://onlinelibrary.wiley.com/doi/abs/10.1002/jcop.20063

Emerson, D., Hopper, E., Kolk, B., Levine, P. A., & Cope, S. (2011). *Overcoming Trauma through Yoga: Reclaiming Your Body* (Illustrated ed.). North Atlantic Books.

Emerson, D., Sharma, R., Chaudhry, S., & Turner, J. (2009). Trauma-sensitive yoga: Principles, practice, and research. *International Journal of Yoga Therapy, 19,* 123–128.

Fay, D. (2017). *Attachment-based yoga and meditation for trauma recovery: Simple, safe, and effective practices for therapy.* W. W. Norton.

Forbes, B. (2011). *Yoga for emotional balance: Simple practices to help relieve anxiety and depression.* Shambhala.

FORGE Forward. (2017, May 6). *Rebecca Campbell -- The World's Messiest Desk* [Video]. YouTube. https://www.youtube.com/watch?v=vdx2E5wArt8

Frye, J., Phadke, S., Bleiweis, R., Buchanan, M. J., Corley, D., ahmed, O., Cokley, R., Durso, L. E., Parsons, C. (2019, October 31). *Transforming the Culture of Power.* Center for American Progress. https://www.americanprogress.org/issues/women/reports/2019/10/31/476588/transforming-culture-power/

Gessel, N. (2018, June 28). *Trauma-informed yoga: When the breath acts as a trigger.* Elephant Journal. https://www.elephantjournal.com/2018/06/trauma-informed-yoga-when-the-breath-acts-as-a-trigger/

Haelle, T. (2020, September 10). Your 'surge capacity' is depleted - it's why you feel awful. Retrieved 2020, from https://elemental.medium.com/your-surge-capacity-is-depleted-it-s-why-you-feel-awful-de285d542f4c

Harris, J. C., Karunaratne, N., & Gutzwa, J. (in press). Effective Modalities for Healing from Campus Sexual Assault: Centering the Experiences of Women of Color Undergraduate Student Survivors. *Harvard Educational Review*

Harris, J. C., & Linder, C. (2017). *Intersections of Identity and Sexual Violence on Campus: Centering Minoritized Students' Experiences.* Stylus Publishing.

Heidt, J. M., Marx, B. P., & Forsyth, J. P. (2005). Tonic immobility and childhood sexual abuse: a preliminary report evaluating the sequela of rape-induced paralysis. *Behaviour Research and Therapy*, *43*(9), 1157–1171. https://doi.org/10.1016/j.brat.2004.08.005

Howard, M. (2013, August 17). *Part III: Trauma training should be mandatory for yoga teachers*. HuffPost. https://www.huffpost.com/entry/yoga-and-healing_b_3451883

James, S. E., Brown, C., & Wilson, I. (2017). 2015 U.S. Transgender Survey: Report on the Experiences of Black Respondents. Washington, DC and Dallas, TX: National Center for Transgender Equality, Black Trans Advocacy, & National Black Justice Coalition.

James, S. E., Herman, J. L., Rankin, S., Keisling, M., Mottet, L., & Anafi, M. (2015). *2015 U.S. transgender survey*. Issuu. https://issuu.com/lgbtagingcenter/docs/usts-full-report-final

Kendall, M. (2020). *Hood feminism: Notes from the women that a movement forgot*. Viking.

Klein, M. C., Heagberg, K., Ashworth, K., & Willis, T. (Eds.). (2020). *Embodied Resilience through Yoga: 30 Mindful Essays About Finding Empowerment After Addiction, Trauma, Grief, and Loss*. Llewellyn Publications.

Lamott, A. (n.d.). Retrieved Spring, 2020, from https://i.redd.it/3by6kdwjrz331.jpg

Lanier, C. (2019, August 2). *Contraindications of pranayama as it applies to trauma survivors*. Embodied Philosophy. https://www.embodiedphilosophy.com/contraindications-of-pranayama-as-it-applies-to-trauma-survivors/

Levine, P. A., Ph.D. (2008). *Healing Trauma: A Pioneering Program for Restoring the Wisdom of Your Body* (New Edition). Sounds True.

Lewis, L. (2021, January 20). Creating a safe training environment for clients who are survivors. *Girls Gone Strong*. https://www.girlsgonestrong.com/blog/articles/creating-a-safe-training-environment-for-clients-who-are-survivors/

Lorde, A. (1982). *Learning from the 60s*. BlackPast. https://www.blackpast.org/african-american-history/1982-audre-lorde-learning-60s/

Macy, R. J., Jones, E., Graham, L. M., & Roach, L. (2018). Yoga for trauma and related mental health problems: A meta-review with clinical and service recommendations. *Trauma, Violence, & Abuse*, *19*(1), 35–57. https://pubmed.ncbi.nlm.nih.gov/26656487/

Marx, B. P., Forsyth, J. P., Gallup, G. G., Fusé, T., & Lexington, J. M. (2008). Tonic immobility as an evolved predator defense: Implications for sexual assault survivors. *Clinical Psychology: Science and Practice*, *15*(1), 74–90. https://doi.org/10.1111/j.1468-2850.2008.00112.x

McCarthy, P., Schiraldi, V., & Shark, M. (2016, October). *Future of Youth Justice: A Community-Based Alternative to the Youth Prison Model*. National Institute of Justice. https://www.ojp.gov/pdffiles1/nij/250142.pdf

Miller, O. (2004, September 2). The Chakra Deck: 50 Cards for Promoting Spiritual and Physical Health (Relax and Rejuvenate): Miller, Olivia, Kaufman, Nicole, Damelio, Michele: 9780811841207: Amazon.com: Books. Retrieved 2020, from https://www.amazon.com/Chakra-Deck-Promoting-Spiritual-Rejuvenate/dp/0811841200

Mitchell, K. S., Dick, A. M., DiMartino, D. M., Smith, B. N., Niles, B., Koenen, K., & Street, A. (2014). A pilot study of a randomized controlled trial of yoga as an intervention for PTSD symptoms in women. *Journal of Traumatic Stress*, *27*, 121–128. https://www.ptsd.va.gov/professional/articles/article-pdf/id42064.pdf

Möller, A., Söndergaard, H. P., & Helström, L. (2017). Tonic immobility during sexual assault - a common reaction predicting post-traumatic stress disorder and severe depression. *Acta Obstetricia et Gynecologica Scandinavica, 96*(8), 932–938. https://doi.org/10.1111/aogs.13174

Munson, M., & Cook-Daniels, L. (2015, September). *Transgender Sexual Violence Survivors: A Self Help Guide to Healing and Understanding.* FORGE. https://forge-forward.org/wp-content/uploads/2020/08/self-help-guide-to-healing-2015-FINAL.pdf

Nagoski, E., & Nagoski, A. (2019). *Burnout: The secret to unlocking the stress cycle.* Ballantine Books.

Nahai, A. (2018). *Trauma to dharma: Transform your pain into purpose.* AnR Books.

National Alliance on Mental Illness. (n.d.) *Types of mental health professionals.* Retrieved Spring, 2020, from https://www.nami.org/About-Mental-Illness/Treatments/Types-of-Mental-Health-Professionals

The National Council for Behavioral Health. (2013, May). *How to Manage Trauma* [Infographic]. https://www.thenationalcouncil.org/wp-content/uploads/2013/05/Trauma-infographic.pdf?daf=375ateTbd56

National Sexual Violence Resource Center. (2011). *National intimate partner and sexual violence survey initial talking points.* https://www.nsvrc.org/publications/NISVS-initial-talking-points

National Sexual Violence Resource Center (NSVRC). (2017). *Building cultures of care: A guide for sexual assault services programs.* https://www.nsvrc.org/publications/nsvrc-publications-guides/building-cultures-care-guide-sexual assault-services-programs

Office for Civil Rights. (2011, April 4). *Dear colleague letter.* https://www2.ed.gov/about/offices/list/ocr/letters/colleague-201104.html

Ogden, P., Minton, K., Pain, C., Siegel, D. J., & Kolk, B. (2006). *Trauma and the body: A sensorimotor approach to psychotherapy (Norton Series on Interpersonal Neurobiology)* W. W. Norton & Company.

Parker, G. (2019, July 14). A yoga therapist shares the truth about trauma. *Yoga Journal.* https://www.yogajournal.com/yoga-101/yoga-therapist-shares-truth-about-trauma

Parker, G. (2020). Restorative yoga for ethnic and race-based stress and trauma. In *Restorative Yoga for Ethnic and Race-Based Stress and Trauma* (p. 90). London: Jessica Kingsley.

Patterson, J. (2020). *The power of breathwork: Simple practices to promote wellbeing.* Fair Winds Press.

Phoenix, O. (2015). *Self care wheel.* http://www.olgaphoenix.com/wp-content/uploads/2015/05/SelfCare-Wheel-Final.pdf

Poore, T., Shulruff, T., & Bein, K. (2013). *Holistic healing services for survivors SASP white paper.* Indiana Criminal Justice Institute. https://resourcesharingproject.org/sites/default/files/Holistic%2BHealing%2BSASP%2BPaper%2BFINAL.pdf

Porges, S. W. (2017). *The pocket guide to the polyvagal theory: The transformative power of feeling safe.* W. W. Norton.

RAINN. (n.d.). *Dissociation.* https://www.rainn.org/articles/dissociation

RAINN.org. (2019). Scope of the problem: StatisticsRAINNORG. Retrieved 2020, from https://www.rainn.org/statistics/scope-problem

Reeves, E. (2015). A synthesis of the literature on trauma-informed care. *Issues in Mental Health Nursing, 36*(9), 698–709.

Remen, R. N. (1996). *Kitchen Table Wisdom: Stories That Heal*. New York, United States: Macmillan Publishers.

Rhodes, A., Spinazzola, J., & van der Kolk, B. (2016). Yoga for adult women with chronic PTSD: A long-term follow-up study. *The Journal of Alternative and Complementary Medicine, 22*(3).

Rosenberg, S. (2017). *Accessing the healing power of the vagus nerve: Self-help exercises for anxiety, depression, trauma, and autism*. North Atlantic Books.

Rozentsvit, I. (2016). The post-traumatic growth: The wisdom of the mind, its clinical and neuropsychoanalytic vicissitudes. *European Psychiatry, 33*(S1), S568-S568. doi:10.1016/j.eurpsy.2016.01.2105

Shah, P. (2020, August 20). *A Primer of the Chakra System*. Chopra. https://chopra.com/articles/what-is-a-chakra

Sidran Institute Traumatic Stress Education & Advocacy. (2018). *Traumatic Stress Disorder Fact Sheet*. Retrieved 2020. https://www.sidran.org/wp-content/uploads/2018/11/Post-Traumatic-Stress-Disorder-Fact-Sheet-.pdf

Siegel, D. J. (1999). *The developing mind: How relationships and the brain interact to shape who we are*. Guilford Publications.

Substance Abuse and Mental Health Services Administration. (2014) *SAMHSA's Concept of Trauma and Guidance for a Trauma-Informed Approach*. HHS Publication No. (SMA) 14-4884. Rockville, MD: Substance Abuse and Mental Health Services Administration. https://ncsacw.samhsa.gov/userfiles/files/SAMHSA_Trauma.pdf.

Substance Abuse and Mental Health Services Administration (SAMHSA). (2013). *Results from the 2012 National Survey on Drug Use and Health: Summary of national findings* (NSDUH Series H-46, HHS Publication No. [SMA] 13-4795). https://www.samhsa.gov/data/sites/default/files/NSDUHresults2012/NSDUHresults2012.pdf

Telles, S. (2012). Managing mental health disorders resulting from trauma through yoga: A review. *Depression Research and Treatment, 2012*, 1–9.

Testa, M., & Dermen, K. H. (1999). The Differential Correlates of Sexual Coercion and Rape. *Journal of Interpersonal Violence, 14*(5), 548–561. https://doi.org/10.1177/088626099014005006

The White House. (2017, January 5). *FACT SHEET: Final It's On Us Summit and Report of the White House*. Retrieved 2020, from https://obamawhitehouse.archives.gov/the-press-office/2017/01/05/fact-sheet-final-its-us-summit-and-report-white-house-task-force-protect

Transgender Sexual Violence Project. (2019, September 30). *Statistics*. Retrieved from Metoomvmt.org website: https://metoomvmt.org/learn-more/statistics/

Treleaven, D. A. (2018). *Trauma-sensitive mindfulness: Practices for safe and transformative healing*. W. W. Norton.

U.S. Department of Defense. (2018, May 1). *DoD Releases Annual Report on Sexual Assault in Military*. Retrieved 2020, from https://www.defense.gov/Explore/News/Article/Article/1508127/dod-releases-annual-report-on-sexual-assault-in-military/

U.S. Department of Education, Office for Civil Rights. (2011, April 4). *Dear colleague letter*. https://www2.ed.gov/about/offices/list/ocr/letters/colleague-201104.html

Walker, H. E., Freud, J. S., Ellis, R. A., Fraine, S. M., & Wilson, L. C. (2019). The Prevalence of Sexual Revictimization: A Meta-Analytic Review. *Trauma, Violence, & Abuse, 20*(1), 67–80. https://doi.org/10.1177/1524838017692364

West, J., Liang, B., & Spinazzola, J. (2017). Trauma sensitive yoga as a complementary treatment for posttraumatic stress disorder: A qualitative descriptive analysis. *International Journal of Stress Management, 24*(2), 173–195. https://doi.org/10.1037/str0000040

Zaleski, K. L., Johnson, D., & Klein, J. (2016). Grounding Judith Herman's trauma theory within interpersonal neuroscience and evidence based practice modalities for trauma treatment. *Smith College Studies in Social Work, 86*(4), 1–17

Zaleski, K. L. (2018). *Understanding and treating military sexual trauma* (2nd ed.). Springer.

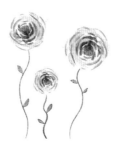

# INDEX

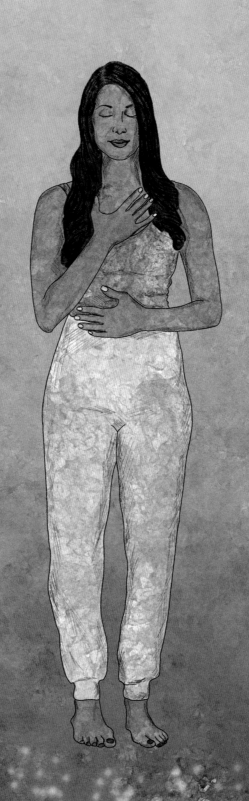

# ABOUT THE AUTHOR

**Zahabiyah (Zabie) Yamasaki**, M.Ed., RYT (she/her), is the Founder of Transcending Sexual Trauma through Yoga which is an organization that offers trauma-informed yoga to survivors, consultation for universities and trauma agencies, and training for healing professionals. Zabie has trained thousands of yoga instructors and mental health professionals and her trauma-informed yoga program and curriculum is now being implemented at over 25 colleges campuses and agencies including the University of California (UC) system, Stanford, Yale, USC, University of Notre Dame, and Johns Hopkins University.

Zabie received her undergraduate in Psychology and Social Behavior and Education at UC Irvine and completed her graduate degree in Higher Education Administration and Student Affairs at The George Washington University. Her work has been highlighted on CNN, NBC, KTLA 5, and The Huffington Post.

Zabie is widely recognized for her intentionality, soulful activism, and passionate dedication to her field. She is a trauma-informed yoga instructor, resilience and well-being educator, and a sought after consultant and keynote speaker. She has worked with thousands of survivors to support them in their healing journey, ground them in their own worthiness and remind them they are inherently whole. Zabie centers survivors in her work, and provides them with tools to help uncover trauma imprints, support the healing process, create balance of the nervous system, and lessen the grip that past experiences of trauma may have on the heart.

She is a survivor, mother, partner, daughter, sister, friend, and activist. She has received countless awards in victim services and leadership, including the Visionary in Victim Services award from one of the largest rape crisis centers in California.

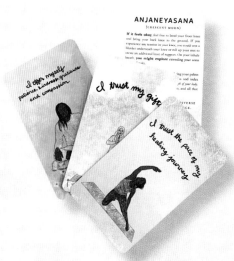
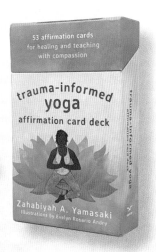
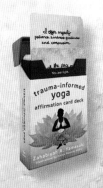